MOLECULAR MECHANISMS OF THE AGING PROCESS AND REJUVENATION

Edited by **Naofumi Shiomi**

Molecular Mechanisms of the Aging Process and Rejuvenation
http://dx.doi.org/10.5772/61700
Edited by Naofumi Shiomi

Contributors
Judit Subirana-Mirete, Jin-Wen Xu, Saverio Gentile, Simon Kaja, Vidhya Rao, Iryna Pishel, Hyun Jeong Park, Miri Kim, Naofumi Shiomi

Published by InTech
Janeza Trdine 9, 51000 Rijeka, Croatia

Publishing Process Manager Andrea Koric
Technical Editor SPi Global
Cover InTech Design team

First published August, 2016
Printed in Croatia

Additional hard copies can be obtained from orders@intechopen.com

Molecular Mechanisms of the Aging Process and Rejuvenation, Edited by Naofumi Shiomi
p. cm.
Print ISBN 978-953-51-2568-6
Online ISBN 978-953-51-2569-3

For EU product safety concerns:
IN TECH d.o.o., Prolaz Marije Krucifikse Kozulić 3, 51000 Rijeka, Croatia,
info@intechopen.com or visit our website at intechopen.com.

Meet the editor

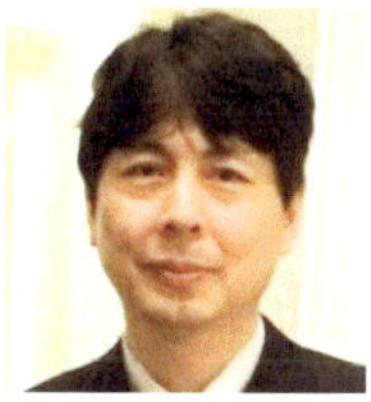

Dr. Naofumi Shiomi studied recombinant yeast and its utilization as a researcher at the Laboratory of Production Technology of Kanena Corporation for 15 years until 1998 and earned his PhD in Engineering from Kyoto University. He now works as a professor at the School of Human Sciences of Kobe College in Japan, where he teaches applied microbiology, biotechnology, and life science in his "Applied Life Science" laboratory. He has studied bioremediation and biomedical science for 17 years at Kobe College and has published more than 40 papers and several book chapters. His recent research has focused on the prevention of obesity and aging.

Contents

Preface

Why do living things gradually senesce? This question is an important theme for human beings, and numerous studies have sought its answer. Some 30 years ago, Brackbarn et al. discovered that telomeres functioned as a clock of cell life, remarkably advancing studies on the molecular mechanisms of aging. As a result, many genes and proteins related to aging have been discovered and their roles elucidated. However, we have not yet answered the main question because of the complicated mechanism of aging in cells. Regarding aging in tissues, many factors such as biologically active substances, signal proteins, hormones, the immune system, and the environment are involved in the process. As such, the complexities of the mechanism make understanding of the fine details difficult. Comprehensive discussion is necessary to clarify the mechanisms underlying aging and rejuvenation.

I therefore proposed to publish this book to obtain a comprehensive assessment of the recent advances in the fields of aging and rejuvenation. In the early parts of this book, the overall aspect of the aging and rejuvenation processes is introduced by the editor, with other researchers expanding on the role of the genes of the circadian clock and ion channel, which, respectively, control the rhythms of cells and calcium ions and decrease those functions due to aging. Techniques capable of improving these functions may provide a novel rejuvenation system.

In the latter chapters, the mechanisms underlying aging and rejuvenation in tissues are introduced. Researchers will describe the aging of skin, the molecular mechanism of skin aging, and the role of certain compounds and oxidative stress in antiaging. We then move on to discussing the role of aging-related molecules in the blood. The results of attempts at rejuvenation by parabiosis between young and old mice or injection of blood components are reviewed, and the possibility of the successful development of antiaging therapy is discussed. Antiaging therapy using blood components may become a realizable and immediately useful procedure for rejuvenation. Finally, we examine novel biomarkers for mild cognitive impairment and Alzheimer's disease, which play an important role in preventing aging in the brain.

I believe that this book will be useful for those studying or developing new drugs to counter the aging process and for students studying aging. Furthermore, it may provide novel ideas on aging and rejuvenation procedures, in addition to supplying important information on available techniques.

I would like to thank Ms. Andrea Koric, Ms. Ivona Lovric, the publishing process managers of the InTech Publishing Group for their great support and assistance throughout the writing and publication process of this book.

Prof. Naofumi Shiomi
School of Human Sciences, Kobe College
Japan

Chapter 1

Introductory Chapter: Recent Studies on Cellular Aging and Rejuvenation

Naofumi Shiomi

Additional information is available at the end of the chapter

http://dx.doi.org/10.5772/63897

1. Introduction

Certain creatures possess the properties of eternal youth and deathlessness. These include Turritopsis (a species of small jellyfish) and planarians. Old Turritopsis starts a degeneration to transform into polyps and thereby achieves a perpetual life cycle [1]. The old cells contained in an old imago change into young cells when the imago transforms into a polyp. The polyp then starts to grow until it reaches the imago stage. As the Turritopsis can repeat this cycle forever, it can be considered to exist in a state of deathlessness. Planarians possess a special property of not growing older. They contain numerous stem cells throughout their bodies and every portion of their body can reproduce [2]. Planarians may therefore be an ageless organism. The property of agelessness is also present in humans. The case of Brooke Greenberg, an American woman who could not grow older after developing highlander syndrome, was the subject of a number of news reports in Japan a few years ago [3]. Moreover, there are several reported cases of female patients who developed highlander syndrome; however, the veracity of these reports is unclear, and the gene that causes the syndrome has not been elucidated. The development of highlander syndrome in human patients suggests that humans might possess the genes that enable the property of eternal youth.

The actualization of eternal youth is a long-held dream, and numerous studies have been performed to elucidate the mechanisms of aging and to achieve eternal youth. Consequently, recent studies have partially elucidated the process of aging and proposed several anti-aging or rejuvenation procedures; however, the studies are currently in the middle stage, and the key elements of the aging process have yet to be elucidated. The purpose of this chapter is to present an overview of the recent topics on cellular aging and rejuvenation to provide an outline of the content in this book. This chapter also complements the chapters that follow; in which researchers introduce topics related to aging and rejuvenation.

2. The mechanisms of cellular aging

2.1. Aging by telomere shortening

Cultured human cells become older through repeated cell division. Cells eventually stop dividing when they reach the critical passage number, the Hayflick limit [4]. Blackburn [5] and Greider discovered that the telomeres function as a clock by marking the passage of time in cells. The molecular mechanism of aging, which is described below [6–8], was elucidated through this discovery.

RNA primer is degraded and exchanged to DNA with DNA polymerase I followed by replication with DNA polymerase III. However, the RNA primer present at the terminal portion of telomeres cannot be exchanged to DNA. As a result, approximately 100 sequence bases are shortened in every replication. The shortening of telomeres acts as a fuse and decides the limit of cell division. The length limit (M1 period) in human fibroblasts is approximately 5 kb, but most cells in elderly humans do not reach the M1 period [9]. Moreover, mouse telomeres are of sufficient length, even in old mice, due to the expression of telomerase. Otherwise, cells in the M1 period can continue to undergo cell division by transforming with T antigen [10]. In such cells, the shortening of telomeres continues, and cell division is finally stopped again by the fusion of mutual terminals (the M2 period) or apoptosis. Telomeres are therefore protected from further shortening by a safe limit (the M1 period).

The pathway from telomere shortening to the cessation of cell division has also been elucidated [7]. A telomere is formed by both double-stranded DNA, which is made by repeated sequences ("TTAGGG" in the mammals), and single-strand DNA (G-tail) of similar sequences that exist at the terminal portion. A telomere has to construct the T-rope structure to avoid degradation by DNA degrading enzymes. This structure gives the first signal to initiate the progression of cell division. The shortening of telomeres causes the obstruction of the T-rope structure and signals certain proteins, including telomeric repeat-binding factor 2 (TRF2), AMP kinase and histone deacetylase, to delay or stop cell division. The detection of the signal by AMP kinase activates p53 and/or p21 proteins and inhibits the work of the cyclin-dependent kinase (CDK) complex. Finally, the inhibition of the CDK complex causes cell division to stop at the Go period, because CDK is a control switch that determines whether cell division should be promoted.

2.2. The effects of mitochondria on the aging process

Mitochondria also have a role in the aging process [11, 12]. Mitochondria produce ATP using the electron transport chain pathway where reactive oxygen species (hydrogen peroxide, hydroxyl radical and hydroperoxyl radical) are produced. Reactive oxygen species are often leaked through the mitochondrial inner membrane, damage DNA, proteins, and lipids. It has been confirmed by the experiments with nematodes [13] that reactive oxygen species promote aging. For instance, the mutation of the mev-1 gene in nematodes was found to result in a shorter life span, because the gene disruption caused a defect in the electron transport chain and an increase in the level of reactive oxygen species. Conversely, a mutation of the age-1 gene in nematodes caused the enhancement of catalase activity which degraded hydrogen peroxide and resulted in a prolonged life span.

Recent studies have suggested an interaction between mitochondrial dysfunction and telomere shortening because of the following process [12, 14, 15]. The shortening of telomeres causes the activation of the p53 protein, the activation of which inhibits the activities of PGC-1α and β, which induce the activation of mitochondria. This inhibition finally causes a decrease in many important mitochondrial activities and the progression of the aging process. On the contrary, an increase in the level of active oxygen species due to mitochondrial dysfunction often causes the oxidation of telomeres; the numerous guanine repeats on telomeres cause them to react easily with oxygen. In telomere DNA, oxidation disturbs the combination of TRF2 with telomere DNAs and the normal T-rope structure, which is the first signal that cell division cannot proceed. Thus, under high concentrations oxygen, the telomeres in human cells are rapidly shortened and cell growth is inhibited.

2.3. The factors promoting the aging process

Studies using both old cells (M1 period) and young cells (Low PDL) have suggested other causes of the aging. When cell fusion occurs between a young cell and an old cell from which the nucleus has been removed, the cell division of the fused cell is inhibited. However, when old cells that were previously treated with a protein synthesis inhibitor are used, growth is not inhibited. Moreover, when the cell membrane of old cells or mRNAs of cells stopped at the Go period, respectively, are injected into younger cells, cell division stops or DNA replication is inhibited. These results suggest that some proteins, mRNAs and/or cell membranes that are present in older cells gradually accumulate with every cell division and promote the aging process. The genes corresponding to such compounds have also been screened [16, 17]. Some genes (gas, gadd, mot1, and hic-5) have been cloned. Unfortunately, they were not the most important genes for controlling the aging process. Recently screening has been performed using RNA, and some promising genes have been identified [18, 19].

2.4. The genes associated with premature senility syndromes

Information that is important for elucidating the aging process in humans can be obtained from the genes that cause premature senility syndrome. Five types of helicases (RecQL1, BLM, WRN RecQL4/RTS, and RecQL5) that untangle DNA chains exist in humans. The change of the proteins to abnormal sequences causes premature senility syndromes [20]. Werner, Bloom, and Rothmund–Thomson syndromes are caused by abnormal structures of the WRN, BLM, and RecQL4/RT proteins, respectively. The WRN protein, which is related to the replication, restoration, transcription, and stabilization of DNA or telomeres, is remarkable. In the case of patients of Werner syndrome, the onset of symptoms occurs after patients stop growing at approximately 10 years of age. In Werner syndrome, the aging process advances much faster than in normal individuals. Patients show normal nerve and immune systems but possess unusual chromosomes. The WRN gene was expected to become a target of aging in normal individuals, because with the exception of the speed at which aging advances, the symptoms are similar to the normal aging process. However, WRN knockout mice do not show premature senility syndrome, whereas WRN and TERC knockout mice do [21]. Further investigation is necessary to improve our understanding of the relationship between WRN and the aging process.

The other remarkable premature senility syndrome is Hutchinson–Gilford progeria syndrome (HGPS), which is caused by partial loss of the lamin A protein [22]. HGPS patients are normal at birth. HGPS develops at 6–18 months of age; the average life span of an HGPS patient is 13 years. Lamin A exists inside a nuclear membrane and supports the structure of the membrane. It is changed to a farnesylated version to perform nuclear translocation, and farnesylated lamin A is related to both the replication and transcription of DNA and signal transduction. The unusual farnesylated lamin A that is found in HGPS patients is called "progerin" [23]. Progerin accumulates and inhibits translocation, and the inhibition causes the aging of cells. In normal individuals, progerin gradually accumulates in the skin cells due to aging. Progerin is therefore a target of treatments to delay the aging process.

3. Realizing cellular rejuvenation

3.1. Rejuvenation by telomerase activation

In humans, although telomerase can make telomeres longer, most types of cells (including fibroblasts, spanchnic cells, and nerve cells) show very low telomerase activity [24]. In contrast, germ and cancer cells, which actively perform cell division, show high telomerase activity and long telomeres. This suggests that the cells may be rejuvenated if telomerase can be activated [25–27].

Studies on the fibroblasts and mice that express telomerase reverse transcriptase (TERT) gene by transformation have supported this hypothesis [28–30]. For example, a human OSMU36-T2 fibroblast showing high telomerase activity was obtained by transforming the TERT gene into an OSMU36 fibroblast. The telomere length and the telomerase activity of OSMU36-T2 were several times higher than those observed in OSMU36 fibroblast, and many characteristics including the cell size, growth rate, and gene expression were similar to those observed in young fibroblasts [28]. Moreover, the life span of a TERT knockout mouse, which was produced by Harvard University, was much shorter (only 6 months) than normal mice due to the rapid shortening of the telomeres. When telomerase was activated in the knockout mice, neurons were formed and rejuvenation was found in some portions [29, 30]. Thus, it may be possible to initiate cellular rejuvenation in individuals as well as cultured cells through the activation of telomerase.

Telomerase activity and telomere length are affected by lifestyle [31, 32]. Researchers at California University group examined the effects of food, exercise, and psychological stress on the telomere length in 35 males [31]. The members of one group continued to consume vegetables as a staple food, to perform adequate exercise and to decrease psychological stress through self-control for 5 years. As a result, their telomeres were longer than the members of the control group. Other researchers investigated the effects of exercise. The results suggested that the athletes who ran more than 40 km every day were 16 years younger in telomere length.

Moreover, telomerase can be activated by some chemical compounds, which are expected to have applications as rejuvenation drugs. For instance, the rate at which telomeres shorten is accelerated by high serum concentrations of cholesterol, because cholesterol hastens cell division. Thus, mononucleosis patients who continuously took statin (an anticholesteremic agent) showed higher telomerase activity and longer telomeres than the patients who did not take statin [33]. Several years ago, a compound named TA-65, which was isolated from the root of the Hedysarum, was screened as a telomerase activating compound [34], and the rejuvenation effect of TA-65 was examined in mice.

As telomerase activity can be controlled by lifestyle and some compounds, the enhancement of telomerase activity may become an effective treatment to promote cellular rejuvenation. However, the enhancement of telomerase activity may also cause the activation or induction of cancer cells, because high telomerase activity is one of the characteristics of cancer cells [35–37]. Further studies to determine whether the activation of telomerase can truly induce a rejuvenation condition without the risk of cancer cell activation will be necessary before it can be used in supplements and drugs.

3.2. Rejuvenation by antioxidants

Leucocytes secrete reactive oxygen species to protect against psychological stress in social life or physical stresses including atmospheric pollutants, UV, and viruses. The excessive production of reactive oxygen species promotes aging (as described in Section 2.2.). Although catalase, superoxide dismutase (SOD), and glutathione peroxydase can remove such reactive oxygen species in humans, catalase, and SOD activities gradually decrease due to aging. Thus, reactive oxygen species cannot be sufficiently removed in elderly individuals. In other words, the aging process can be delayed or remediated if the excessive production of reactive oxygen species is prevented.

Antioxidants, such as vitamins and polyphenols, are effective in removing active oxygen species, and their anti-aging effects have been studied for many years [38, 39]. The studies suggest that the oxidation of cultured cells can be inhibited by antioxidants and that mice that continuously took antioxidants showed lower oxidation and a longer life span than controls. Recent studies in humans, however, suggested that the anti-aging effects are doubtful. For example, in experiments in which healthy human subjects took β-carotene or vitamins for a long period of time, the ratio of depth was not decreased. Certain amounts or components of antioxidants may be required to make the effects of antioxidants prominent in humans.

3.3. Rejuvenation by anti-aging hormones

Anti-aging hormones have remarkable potential as anti-aging or rejuvenation treatments. There are several candidate compounds, including klotho, sirtuin, Bach1, Clk-1, and polyamines [40–46]. The klotho gene is mainly expressed in the nervous system to control the calcium concentration in blood; klotho works as a controller of homeostasis, although the precise work of the protein has not been sufficiently elucidated [40, 41]. Klotho knockout mice develop many symptoms related to aging, such as arteriosclerosis, osteoporosis, motor impairment and have a shortened life span. Conversely, klotho knock-in mice have a life span that is several years longer [42]. Thus, klotho is a promising target in rejuvenation.

Histone deacetylases (sirtuin) is another candidate protein [43, 44]. Sirtuin works as an energy economizing hormone to prolong the life span. Sirtuin 1, 6 and 7 knockout mice showed faster aging and a shorter life span. Hibernation, which represents a state of extreme energy limitation, extended the life spans of yeasts, rematodes, and mice. One reason for the prolongation of the life span is that the amount of excess active oxygen is decreased by the energy limitation; thus, the promotion of the aging process by undesirable oxidation is inhibited. Another cause is the activity of sirtuin. Sirtuin 2 is activated by the decrease of NAD, which is caused by energy limitation. The activation of sirtuin 2 increases the deacetylation of histones to silence the genes, and the economizing of energy prolongs life span.

The following monkey experiments were performed to estimate the action of sirtuin in relation to energy limitation. The Wisconsin National Primate Research Center examined the effects of calorie restriction on 76 rhesus monkeys. The monkeys that had were fed low-calorie food (a 30% calorie reduction) looked much younger and showed a longer life span than control members (100% calorie) [47]. However, a similar experiment by the NIA in the United States in 2012 suggested the reverse results [48]. Therefore, further discussion is necessary to confirm the relationship between anti-aging and energy limitation.

Resveratrol has been screened as a compound that is effective for enhancing the expression of the sirtuin gene [49]. When resveratrol was given to mice that had been fed a high-calorie diet, some of the factors of aging were inhibited, and the activities of AMPK and PGC-1α were enhanced; however, the anti-aging were insufficient. If compounds that can more effectively enhance the sirtuin gene are discovered, they will become a prominent anti-aging hormone.

Polyamines also show remarkable characteristics. Polyamines, such as spermine, spermidine, and putrescine, are essential for the growth of mammals and play important roles in cell division and differentiation; however, their precise action has not been sufficiently elucidated [50, 51]. In most cells of the human body, the concentrations are maintained at low levels. They are only found at high levels in cells that are actively working, such as testicular cells and cancer cells. The amounts of polyamines in those cells are especially increased before DNA synthesis; the growth rate in cancer cells increases in proportion to the amount of polyamine that is added to the medium. Polyamines are therefore related to the activation of cells.

Some studies suggest that polyamines function as an anti-aging hormone. The addition of polyamines to fibroblasts enhanced the expression of genes related to aging [20], and mice that were contentiously fed a diet containing a high concentration of polyamine appeared much younger and had a longer life span than mice that were fed a diet without polyamine [52]. Other researchers, who had studied the relationship between *Lactobacillus bifidus* and life span, suggested that the life span of mice was prolonged by the polyamines that were produced by *L. bifidus* cells [53, 54]. The amounts of spermine and spermidine in humans gradually decrease due to aging, and the concentration of polyamines in the blood can easily be increased by eating foods, such as soy beans. Thus, polyamines may also be useful as supplements for anti-aging or rejuvenation.

4. Conclusion

In this chapter, the author focused on cellular aging and rejuvenation. Recent studies have gradually elucidated the aging process and have suggested that telomerase, the mitochondria and other components (RNAs and proteins) are involved in the aging process. However, these studies are ongoing. Moreover, studies on the aging process have identified several anti-aging compounds that can activate telomerase (TA-65), inactivate reactive oxygen species (anti-oxidants) and work as anti-aging hormones (klotho, sirtuin, resveratrol, and polyamine). In the near future, these compounds and/or other compounds with greater effects may become prominent drugs for anti-aging and rejuvenation.

Research into regeneration with the use of iPS cells is recently showing remarkable progress. Although the topic was not introduced in this chapter, the regeneration of cutaneous and nerve tissues or internal organs using regeneration medicine will be another means of realizing rejuvenation. Researchers studying anti-aging will have to watch the progress of both regeneration medicine and cellular rejuvenation research.

Author details

Naofumi Shiomi*

Address all correspondence to: shiomi@mail.kobe-c.ac.jp

Department of Human Sciences, Kobe College, Hyogo, Japan

References

[1] Kubota S. Repeating rejuvenation in turritopsis, an immortal hydrozoan. (Cnidaria, Hydrozoa). Biogeography (2011); 13:101–103.

[2] Perrigue P.M., Najbauer J., Jozwiak A.A., Barciszewski J., Aboody K.S., Barish M.E.. Planarians as a model of aging to study the interaction between stem cells and senescent sells in vivo. Pathobiology of Aging & Age Related Diseases 2015;5:30052.

[3] Brooke Greenberg. https://en.wikipedia.org/wiki/Brooke Greenberg.

[4] Shay J.W., Wright W.E. Hayflick. His limit, and cellular ageing. Nature Reviews. Mollecular Cell Biology 2000; 1(1):72–6.

[5] Greider C.W., Blackburn E.H. Identification of a specific telomere terminal transferase activity in tetrahymena extracts. Cell 1985,43(2 Pt 1):405–13.

[6] Grach A. Telomere shortening mechanisms. In: Stuart D. (ed) The mechanism of DNA replication, Rijeca, InTech; 2013.

[7] Becker T., Haferkamp S. Molecular mechanisms of cellular senescence. In: Wang Z., Inuzuka H. (ed) Senescence and senescence-related disorders, Rijeca, InTech; 2013.

[8] Davinelli S., Vasto S., Caruso C., Zella D., Scapagnini G. Molecular biomarkers of aging. In: Nagata T. (ed) Senescence, Rijeca, InTech; 2012.

[9] Aikata H., Takaishi H., Kawakami Y., Takahashi S., Kitamoto M., Nakanishi T., Nakamura Y., Shimamoto F., Kajiyama G., Ide T. Telomere reduction in human liver tissues with age and chronic inflammation. Experimental Cell Research 2000;256(2): 578–82.

[10] Shay J.W., Wright W.E., Werbin H. Defining the molecular mechanisms of human cell immortalization. Biochimica Biophysica Acta. 1991;1072(1):1–7.

[11] Lauria A., Pompilioa G., Capogrossi M.C. The mitochondrial genome in aging and senescence. Ageing Research Reviews 2014;18:1–15.

[12] Wiley C.D., Velarde M.C., Lecot P., Liu S., Sarnoski E.A., Freund A., Shirakawa K., Lim H.W., Davis S.S., Ramanathan A., Gerencser A.A., Verdin E., Campisi J. Mitochondrial dysfunction induces senescence with a distinct secretory phenotype. Cell Metabolism 2016: 23(2):303–314.

[13] Honda Y., Honda S. Oxidative stress and life span determination in the nematode *Caenorhabditis elegans*. Annals of New York Academy of Sciences 2002;959:466–74.

[14] Finkel T. Telomerases and mitochondrial function. Circulation Research 2011; 108:903–904.

[15] Sahin E., DePinho R.A. Axis of ageing: telomeres, p53 and mitochondria. Nature Reviews. Molecullar Cell Biology 2012;13(6):397–404.

[16] Sten G.H., Atkins L. Membrane-associated inhibitor of DNA synthesis in senescent human diploid fibroblasts: characterization and comparison to quiescent cell inhibitor. Proceedings of National Academy of United States of America 1986;83:9030–9034.

[17] Lumpkin Jr C.K., McClung J.K., Pereira-Smith O.M., Smith J.R. Existence of high abundance antiproliferative mRNA's in senescent human diploid fibroblasts. Science 1986; 232(4748): 393–395.

[18] Chichinadze K, Tkemaladze D., Lazarashvili A. New class of RNA and centrosomal hypothesis of cell aging. Advances in Gerontology 2012;25(1):23–28.

[19] Gheorghe M., Snoeck M., Emmerich M., Bäck T., Goeman J.J., Raz V. Major aging-associated RNA expressions change at two distinct age-positions. BMC Genomics. 2014;15:132.

[20] Bennett R.J., Keck J.L. Structure and function of RecQ DNA helicases. Critical Reviews in Biochemistry and Molecular Biology. 2004;39(2):79–97.

[21] Chang S., Multani A.S., Cabrera N.G, Naylor M.L., Laud P., Lombard D, Pathak S., Guarente L., DePinho R.A. Essential role of limiting telomeres in the pathogenesis of Werner syndrome. Nature Genetics 2004;36(8):877–882.

[22] Brassard J.A., Fekete N., Garnier A., Hoesli C.A. Hutchinson-Gilford progeria syndrome as a model for vascular aging. Biogerontology. 2016;17(1):129–145.

[23] Chojnowski A., Ong P.F., Wong E.S., Lim J.S., Mutalif R.A., Navasankari R., Dutta B., Yang H., Liow Y.Y., Sze S.K., Boudier T., Wright G.D., Colman A., Burke B., Stewart C.L, Dreesen O. Progerin reduces LAP2α-telomere association in Hutchinson-Gilford Progeria. Elife. 2015;4: e07759.

[24] Kim N.W., Piatyszek M.A., Prowse K.R., Harley C.B., West M.D., Ho P.L., Coviello G.M., Wright W.E., Weinrich S.L., Shay J.W. Specific Association of human telomerase activity with immortal cells and cancer. Science. 1994;266(5193):2011–2015.

[25] Boccardi V., Herbig U. Telomerase gene therapy: a novel approach to combat aging. EMBO Mol Med. 2012;4(8):685–687.

[26] Bernardes de Jesus B., Blasco M.A. Potential of telomerase activation in extending health span and longevity. Current Opinion in Cell Biology 2012;24(6):739–743.

[27] Zhou J., Ding D., Wang M., Cong Y.S. Telomerase reverse transcriptase in the regulation of gene expression. BMB Reports 2014;47(1):8–14.

[28] Shiomi N., Watanabe K. Effects of telomere length on the rejuvenation of cells. Proceedings of 7th Annual Meeting of the Society for Biotechnology, Japan 2015.

[29] Jaskelioff M., Muller F.L., Paik J.H., Thomas E., Jiang S., Adams A.C., Sahin E., Kost-Alimova M., Protopopov A., Cadiñanos J., Horner J.W., Maratos-Flier E., Depinho R.A. Telomerase reactivation reverses tissue degeneration in aged telomerase-deficient mice. Nature 2011;469(7328):102–106.

[30] Tomás-Loba A., Flores I., Fernández-Marcos P.J., Cayuela M.L., Maraver A., Tejera A., Borrás C., Matheu A., Klatt P., Flores J.M., Viña J., Serrano M., Blasco M.A. Telomerase reverse transcriptase delays aging in cancer-resistant mice. Cell 2008;135(4):609–622.

[31] Fernandez E. Lifestyle changes may lengthen telomeres, a measure of cell aging. Diet, Meditation, Exercise Can Improve Key Element of Immune Cell Aging, UCSF Scientists Report 2013.

[32] Mitchell C., Hobcraft J., McLanahan S.S., Siegel S.R., Berg A., Brooks-Gunn J., Garfinkel I., Notterman D. Social disadvantage, genetic sensitivity, and children's telomere length. Proceedings of the National Academy of Science in United State of America 2014;111(16):5944–5949.

[33] Saliques S., Teyssier J.R., Vergely C., Lorgis L., Lorin J., Farnier M., Donzel A., Sicard P., Berchoud J., Lagrost A.C., Touzery C., Ragot S., Cottin Y., Rochette L., Zeller M.

Circulating leukocyte telomere length and oxidative stress: a new target for statin therapy. Atherosclerosis 201;219(2):753–760.

[34] Reichert S., Bize P., Arrivé M., Zahn S., Massemin S., Criscuolo F. Experimental increase in telomere length leads to faster feather regeneration. Experimental Gerontology 2014;52:36–38.

[35] Ding D., Zhou J., Wang M., Cong Y.S. Implications of Telomere-independent activities of telomerase reverse transcriptase in human cancer. FEBS Journal 2013;280(14):3205–3211.

[36] Bernardes de Jesus B., Vera E., Schneeberger K., Tejera A.M., Ayuso E., Bosch F., Blasco M.A. Telomerase gene therapy in adult and old mice delays aging and increases longevity without increasing cancer. EMBO Molecular Medicine 2012;4(8):691–704.

[37] de Jesus B.B., Schneeberger K., Vera E., Tegera A., Harley C.B., Blasco M.A. The Telomerase Activator, TA-65®, Elongates short telomeres and increases health span of adult/old mice without increasing cancer incidence. Aging Cell 2011; 10(4): 604–621.

[38] Fusco D., Colloca G., Lo Monaco M.R. Cesari M. Effects of antioxidant supplementation on the aging process. Clinical Interventions in Aging 2007;2(3):377–387.

[39] Poljsak B., Milisav I. Aging, Oxidative stress and antioxidants. In: Morales-González J.A. (ed) Oxidative stress and chronic degenerative diseases—a role for antioxidants, Rijeka, InTech; 2013.

[40] Nabeshima Y. Klotho: A fundamental regulator of aging. Ageing Research Review 2002;1(4):627–638.

[41] Kuro-o M. Klotho and the aging process. Korean Journal of Internal Medicine 2011; 26(2): 113–122.

[42] Kuro-o M., Matsumura Y., Aizawa H., Kawaguchi H., Suga T., Utsugi T., Ohyama Y., Kurabayashi M., Kaname T., Kume E., Iwasaki H., Iida A., Shiraki-Iida T., Nishikawa S., Nagai R., Nabeshima Y.I. Mutation of the mouse klotho gene leads to a syndrome resembling ageing. Nature 1997;390:45–51.

[43] Wątroba M., Szukiewicz D. The role of sirtuins in aging and age-related diseases. Advances in Medical Sciences 2015;61(1):52–62.

[44] Poulose N., Raju R.. Sirtuin regulation in aging and injury. Biochimica et Biophysica Acta 2015;1852(11):2442–2455.

[45] Stepanyan Z., Hughes B., Cliche D.O., Camp D., Hekimi S. Genetic and molecular characterization of CLK-1/mCLK1, A conserved determinant of the rate of aging. Experimental Gerontology 2006;41(10):940–951.

[46] Igarashi K, Ota K, Nakame A. Regulation of cellular senescence by Bach1. Nihon Rinsho 2009;67(7):1423–1428.

[47] Colman R.J., Anderson R.M., Johnson S.C. Kastman E.K., Kosmatka K.J., Beasley T.M., Allison D.B., Cruzen C., Simmons H.A., Kemnitz J.W., Weindruch R. Caloric Restriction delays disease onset and mortality in rhesus monkeys. Science 2009;325(5937):201–204.

[48] Mattison J.A., Roth G.S., Beasley T.M., Tilmont E.M., Handy A.M., Herbert R.L., Longo D.L., Allison D.B., Young J.E., Bryant M., Barnard D., Ward W.F., Qi W., Ingram D.K., de Cabo R. Impact of caloric restriction on health and survival in rhesus monkeys from the NIA Study. Nature. 2012;489(7415):318–21.

[49] Baur J.A., Pearson K.J., Price N.L. Jamieson H.A., Lerin C., Kalra A., Prabhu V.V., Allard J.S., Lopez-Lluch G., Lewis K., Pistell P.J., Poosala S., Becker K.G., Boss O., Gwinn D., Wang M., Ramaswamy S., Fishbein K.W., Spencer R.G., Lakatta E.G., Le Couteur D., Shaw R.J., Navas P., Puigserver P., Ingram D.K., de Cabo R., Sinclair D.A. Resveratrol improves health and survival of mice on a high-calorie diet. Nature 2006;444(7117):337–342.

[50] Minois N., Carmona-Gutierrez D., Madeo F. Polyamines in aging and disease. Aging (Albany NY) 2011;3(8):716–732.

[51] Pegg A.E. Mammalian polyamine metabolism and function. UBMB Life 2009;61(9):880–894.

[52] Soda K. Polyamines. Nippon Shokuhin Kagaku Kogaku Kaishi 2014; 61(12): 607–624

[53] Linsalata M., Russo F., Berloco P., Caruso M.L., Matteo G.D., Cifone M.G., Simone C.D., Ierardi E., Di Leo A. The influence of *Lactobacillus brevis* on ornithine decarboxylase activity and polyamine profiles in *Helicobacter pylori*-infected *Gastric mucosa*. Helicobacter 2004;9(2):165–172.

[54] Matsumoto M., Kurihara S., Kibe R., Ashida H., Benno Y. Longevity in mice is promoted by probiotic-induced suppression of colonic senescence dependent on upregulation of gut bacterial polyamine production. PLoS One. 2011;6(8):e23652.

Chapter 2

Circadian Clock Gene Regulation in Aging and Drug Discovery

Yufeng Li, Yanqi Dang, Shuang Ling and
Jin-Wen Xu

Additional information is available at the end of the chapter

http://dx.doi.org/10.5772/63184

Abstract

The circadian clock is an endogenous timer in prokaryotes and mammals. Resting and adjusting the internal clock can assist in pacing the daily routine. Growing evidence indicates that the circadian clock and aging process are closely associated. The disruption of the circadian clock leads to accelerated aging and increased incidence of various diseases. In particular, elderly people are more vulnerable and have a higher risk of diseases than do young people. In this study, we reviewed studies on aging and circadian rhythms over the last decade, with a focus on circadian clock gene regulation in aging and drug discovery for targeting the circadian clock in diseases.

Keywords: Bmal1, clock, circadian clock genes, aging, drug discovery

1. Introduction

Circadian rhythms affect almost all daily activity behavioral patterns, physiology, and gene expression. Circadian rhythms indicate the appropriate time for various activities, such as consuming food and mating, and gradually form the circadian clock [1]. The circadian clock is an internal timekeeping system, which facilitates adaptation to the external world in anticipation of daily environmental changes. A 24-h circadian rhythm pattern has been observed in almost all cells [2]. Circadian clocks coordinate external day and night cycles with diverse environmental and metabolic stimuli. However, a disrupted circadian clock causes various diseases, such as insomnia, diabetes, cancer, and metabolic syndrome [3]. The ability of the brain timing system and function of circadian rhythm-regulating genes decline with age. The disruption of circadian rhythms disrupts the coordination among body systems. Aging damages body homeostasis and results in a subhealth status [4]. Consequently, the systems of elderly people are more vulnerable than those of young people [5]. The disruption of circadian rhythms adversely affects the aging process and increases the risk of diseases. A set of circadian clock genes form negative feedback loops that can regulate transcription, with a 24-h circadian oscillation [4, 6]. The circadian function significantly affects the aging process. Chronic destructions of the circadian function are associated with the occurrence of various age-related diseases, such as cancer and premature aging. Therefore, studies are warranted to determine how the circadian clock genes orchestrate interactions between the internal physiology and the aging progress.

In this study, we reviewed studies within the last decade on aging and circadian rhythms and the mechanism underlying the maintenance of biological processes by the circadian clock, with a focus on circadian clock gene regulation in aging and antiaging drug discovery.

2. Circadian clock

2.1. Structure of the circadian system

Living systems possess an exquisite internal biological clock, and the major function of which is to regulate the daily sleep–wake cycle [7]. The circadian clock follows a rhythm of approximately 24 h and ensures accurate adaptation to external daily rhythms through a powerful endogenous timing system [8]. The circadian clock also drives numerous molecular and cellular processes by generating oscillations. Virtually, all body cells have an autonomous circadian clock [9, 10], which is composed of a central clock existing in the suprachiasmatic nucleus (SCN) neuron and peripheral clocks. Clock, Bmal1 (brain and muscle ARNT-like protein-1), Pers, and Crys constitute a set of circadian oscillation genes in mammals [11].

2.1.1. Suprachiasmatic nucleus

The central circadian clock, located in the SCN of the anterior hypothalamus, is the primary circadian pacemaker [12]. The SCN comprises a network of approximately 20,000 neurons. Each neuron is considered to have an oscillator of the autonomous circadian clock. As the neurons are joined and oscillated in a consistent manner [13], the SCN neuron can generate an autonomous circadian clock similar to other cells [14, 15]. The SCN as the primary circadian pacemaker regulates independent gene expressions through neuronal firing [16].

The retina captures optical signals and transmits signals to the SCN (**Figure 1**) [17]. SCN neurons organize coupling mechanisms that ensure their synchronization even in darkness [18]. SCN neurons change the gene expression levels by converting electrical information into chemical information [16]. Neuronal firing frequency can synchronize the other cells of the body with rhythmic changes [19]. The central clock is controlled by external signals; food and light are the strongest signals affecting the clock (**Figure 1**). Once synchronized, the central clock consequently mediates the synchronization of the peripheral clocks through signaling [20].

Moreover, lability and plasticity of the phase in the intrinsic period are two critical functions of the central clock [21]. As the phase is labile, the length of the intrinsic period leads to different phases [22]. The waveform of the SCN amplitude is mainly related to the light cycle. The waveform is narrow with a high amplitude in short photoperiods, whereas it is broader with a low amplitude in long photoperiods. The circadian waveform in SCN oscillation is strong correlated with the SCN and behavioral rhythms [23].

2.1.2. *Peripheral clocks*

Peripheral and central clocks have been discovered in various tissues. One study reported the ubiquity of peripheral clock and its mechanism in both SCN and other cells [24]. Another study reported that cultured SCN cells maintained a firm rhythmic pattern through photoreception, also expressed in many organs, such as the liver, lungs, and kidneys [25]. In addition, numerous mammalian peripheral tissues exhibit circadian oscillation; consequently, oscillations are suppressed when the SCN is absent [9]. Thus, a delayed feedback loop originally associating the same components is considered to be composed of the rhythm-generating molecular circuitry, which is constructed by both SCN and peripheral cells [16]. Several pivotal physiological functions are influenced by light–dark oscillations in peripheral organs (**Figure 1**), including the heart, liver, lung, kidney, and skeletal muscles [26].

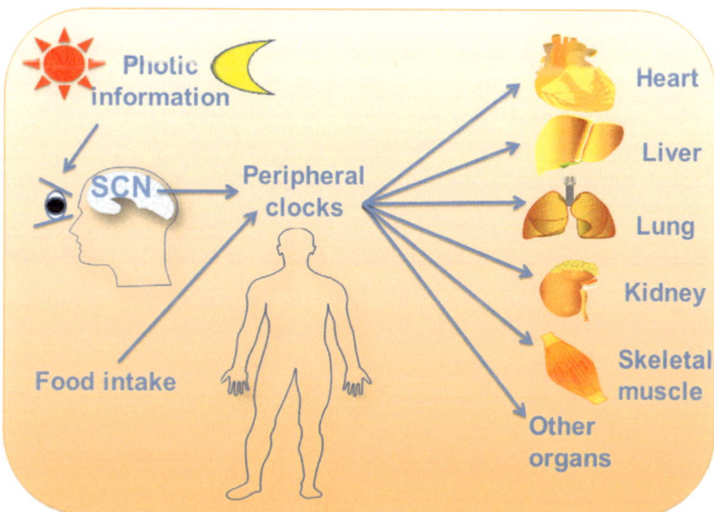

Figure 1. Structure of the circadian system. The retina captures photic information and transmits signals to the SCN. Food and light transmit signals to the peripheral clock.

Local peripheral oscillators can be synchronized by neuronal signals and stimulating hormones. The SCN sends signals to all body systems, coordinating the feeding fasting cycles [27, 28]. Although the SCN functions as the master synchronizer of the entire system, food intake can disrupt the control in peripheral clocks. A change in the feeding schedule alters the phase in the central and peripheral clocks in the liver [29]. Moreover, light information is transmitted to the adrenal gland, liver, and pancreas by the SCN, which distributes a rhythmic signal to all tissues of the peripheral organs [30]. The central neural and peripheral tissues maintain the normal neurological and metabolic homeostasis in the sleep–wake cycle [31]. The endogenous mechanism of oscillation in peripheral cells is a gene regulatory network to generate sustained oscillations. A group of genes forms the core network of the mammalian circadian clock, which can function even in the absence of external inputs in individual cells [32]. Numerous signaling pathways participate in the phase entrainment of peripheral clocks and warrant additional studies.

2.2. Circadian clock and diseases

The circadian clock regulates the sleep–wake cycle, metabolism, hormone secretion, and other physiological processes. A recent study suggested that chronic circadian disruption is deleterious to health and causes myocardial infarction, sudden cardiac death, and aortic aneurysm rupture risk [33]. Circadian dysregulation has extensive consequences not only on glucose control but also on inflammation. REV–ERBα and retinoid-related orphan receptors (RORs), which are downstream proteins of the signaling pathway, can affect adipogenesis and thrombosis through circadian clock regulation. This study indicates that metabolic and circadian pathways, which involve the nuclear receptor superfamily, are associated to the central node [34].

Circadian rhythm and sleep disorders lead to an increased incidence of metabolic syndrome [35]. Chronic sleep curtailment may affect the increase in the prevalence of diabetes and obesity. The effect may change glucose metabolism by reducing energy consumption [36]. Hypothalamic–pituitary–thyroid axis rhythms are endocrine rhythms and are accurately governed by the circadian system [37]. Evidence suggests that a seasonal change in thyroid hormone availability in the hypothalamus, and pituitary gland is a crucial element [38]. Sex-differentiated circadian timing systems exist in the hypothalamic–pituitary–gonadal (HPG) axis, the hypothalamic–adrenal–pituitary (HPA) axis, and sleep-arousal systems [39]. When various stressors appear, the HPA axis adjusts the circadian rhythms of the peripheral clocks through the glucocorticoid receptor [40]. In addition, the female HPG axis is regulated by a molecular clock in gonadotropin secretion because it relates to the timing of gonadotropin secretion in ovulation and parturition [41]. The circadian timing system and estradiol sensitive neural circuits driving the HPG axis functioning include gonadotropin-releasing hormone secretion and preovulatory luteinizing hormone [42].

Moreover, a strong association exists between the circadian clock and hormone secretion. The human placenta synthesizes the melatonin-regulating circadian system of many tissues, and the unusual secretion adversely affects fetal and maternal health [43]. The circadian system, which is composed of a family of clock genes, also regulates hormonal production and activity [44]. Maternal melatonin is a circadian signal for oscillating the fetal SCN clock. However, maternal melatonin probably cannot control the adrenal gland [45]; therefore, the circadian clock system affects the fetus during embryonic development.

Adequate sleep is crucial for maintaining the function of circadian rhythms. The lack of sleep disrupts circadian rhythms. Impaired endocrine and physiological circadian rhythms affect the quantity of immune cells [46]. Circadian oscillations can mediate cognitive performance through sleep. However, it cannot work correctly in case of the environmental disturbance of the clock, including shift work and schedules [47]. Circadian systems are disrupted through inadequate melatonin secretion, and the altered clock gene expression can cause human metabolic syndrome and cardiovascular diseases [35].

3. Circadian clock gene regulation in aging

Circadian oscillations regulate transcription by using a set of genes, thus establishing an autoregulatory feedback loop. A study reported that circadian gene expression is widespread through the body [19]. Animal studies have revealed that a disrupted circadian clock function accelerated the development of aging phenotypes. The temporal precision of circadian system is lost with advancing age. Growing evidence indicates that aging is affected by circadian clocks. Circadian clocks can change gene expression, physiological functions, and daily cycles. The circadian system leads to various age-related pathologies and exhibits a weak precision with advancing age. The aged SCN shows changes in the expression of vasoactive intestinal polypeptide [48]. Circadian rhythms of the electrical activity are decreased [49]. When a young SCN is transplanted into aged animals, the behavioral rhythms functioning in locomotion is improved [50]. These studies indicate that the SCN is crucial to improve the age-related circadian system, which may be deteriorated in aged individuals.

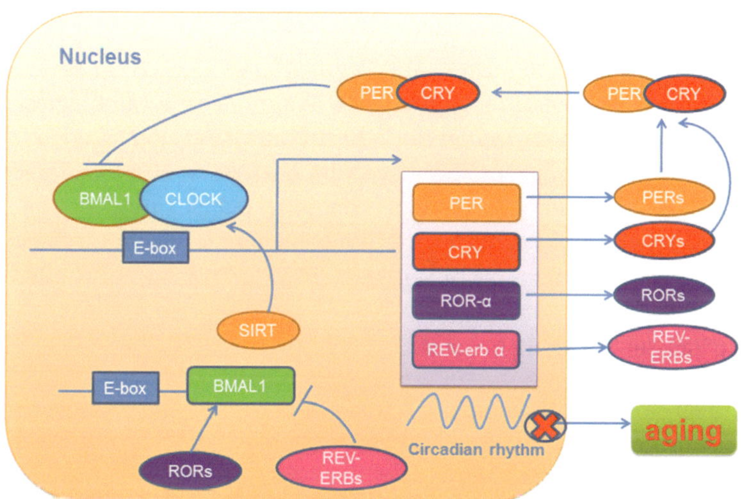

Figure 2. Circadian clock gene regulation in aging.

Bmal1 and clock activate the expression of period (Per), cryptochrome (Cry), RORα, and REV–ERBα. The negative elements of the clock PER and CRY proteins, which are associated with Clock–Bmal1 at E-box sites, enter the nucleus. REV–ERBα competes with each other for their binding DNA in the Bmal1 promoter, and the expression of Bmal1 is repressed.

3.1. Effects of Bmal1 genes on the aging process

Bmal1 belongs to the family of the basic helix–loop–helix (bHLH)–PAS domain containing transcription factors [51]. Bmal1 is a transcriptional factor and major component of the circadian clock; it plays a critical role in accelerating aging and the development of age-related pathologies. Bmal1 as the core clock gene regulates the expression of other circadian clock genes, which affects the physiological circadian rhythm [52]. Bmal1 deficiency has been shown to significantly shorten lifespan and accelerate senescence. *Bmal1*$^{-/-}$ mice have a shorter lifespan and exhibit cataracts, organ shrinkage, and other symptoms of premature aging [53].

Bmal1 may be directly associated with premature aging and reduced lifespan. Recent studies have reported a significantly weakened function of circadian rhythms in aged animals. The disturbances in circadian rhythms may cause thrombosis, a critical result of age-related cardiovascular diseases. Genetic ablation of the gene Bmal1 gene in mice significantly elevates the circulating von Willebrand factor, fibrinogen, and PAI-1 [54]. Bmal1 regulates BDH1 and PIK3R1; thus, Bmal1 affects metabolism, cell signaling, and the contractile function of the heart. Bmal1 predicts impairments in ketone body metabolism and depressing glucose utilization in the hearts of cardiomyocyte-specific Bmal1-knockout mice [55].

Bmal1 is crucial for regulating oxidative stress. Oxidative stress maintains reactive oxygen species (ROS) homeostasis and senescence through the hypoxia-inducible factor-mediated pathway. *Bmal1*$^{-/-}$ cells do not induce replicative senescence but rather stress-induced senescence. Stress-induced senescence causes cell and organ aging [56]. A recent study revealed a significantly decreased rhythmic function in aged animals. The study reported that the activity of the mammalian target of rapamycin complex 1 pathway is controlled by the circadian clock through Bmal1-dependent mechanisms. This regulation evidenced an association between aging and metabolism [57]. Bmal1 in the heart also determines the pathological consequences of the chronic disruption of the circadian clock. *Bmal1*$^{-/-}$ mice develop dilated cardiomyopathy with aging and decreased cardiac performance with changes in titin [58]. In addition, Bmal1 controls the blood coagulation pathway by changing platelet numbers and altering the vascular function. This control results from arterial and venous thrombogenicity by attenuating nitric oxide and anticoagulant factor synthesis [59].

3.2. Effects of Clock on the aging process

Clock is a circadian clock protein similar to Bmal1 and is a transcription factor of the circadian system. Bmal1 and Clock have different functions in modulating the biological function. The deficiency of Clock does not induce any significant age-related changes in organs and tissues; however, they are affected in *Bmal1*$^{-/-}$ mice [60]. The results of Clock and Bmal1 deficiency in physiology are different. Clock encodes a novel bHLH–PAS domain protein of transcription factors [61, 62]. Clock is a unique gene with various features, including DNA binding, protein dimerization, and domain activation [62]. Clock is widely recognized to have circadian functions. The deficiency of the Clock protein significantly affects longevity. The aging of Clock-deficient mice results in a higher rate of pathologies, cataracts, and dermatitis than that of wild-type mice [60].

http://dx.doi.org/10.5772/63184

When Clock is a mutant gene, the pattern of circadian gene expression loses circadian behavior and is disrupted [61, 62]. While Clock in mice is knocked out, the robust circadian rhythms in spontaneous activity are still expressed [63]. Bmal1 forms a heterodimer as the transcriptionally active complex to drive circadian rhythmicity in Clock-deficient animals [64]. In addition, neuronal PAS domain protein 2 functionally replaces the Clock activity in Clock-deficient mice [65]. Age-related circadian changes are caused by both wild-type and heterozygous Clock mutants [66]. Clock–Bmal1 complex activate the transcription of other genes with E-box elements in their promoters [67]. The dimers translocate to the nucleus and obstruct the Clock–Bmal1 complex, thereby hindering the additional transcription of the other genes [68] and ultimately leading Clock and Bmal1 to increase Per transcription and restart the cycle [69]. Clock, as the core component of circadian transcription, operates in complex with another protein. Clock deficiency was shown to cause age-related cataracts [60]. Clock-deficient mice lose body weight, relative organ weight, or ectopic calcification during aging. These mice maintain behavioral rhythms, indicating that peripheral circadian oscillators require Clock [70].

3.3. Effects of the Clock–Bmal1 complex on the aging process

In animals, a transcription–translation loop that revolves around the transcription factors Clock and Bmal1 forms circadian oscillators. The core positive element of the clock is Clock–Bmal1, which is the heterodimeric transcription factor output of circadian locomotor cycles [71]. The negative elements of the clock PER and CRY proteins, associated with Clock–Bmal1 at E-box sites, enter the nucleus [64, 72] (**Figure 2**). The transcriptional activity of Clock–Bmal1 is suppressed by recruiting the SIN3–histone deacetylase (HDAC) complex and preventing transcriptional termination [72, 73]. Histone acetyltransferases (HATs) and HDACs generate rhythms in histone acetylation and the circadian rhythms [74]. Mixed-lineage leukemia protein-1, a H3K4 methyltransferase, has a nonredundant role in the circadian oscillator [75]. The Jumonji C domain-containing H3K4me3 demethylase family and AT-rich interaction domain-containing histone lysine demethylase 1a form a Clock–Bmal1 complex; the complex is then recruited to the Per2 promotor, simultaneously enhancing transcription by Clock–Bmal1 [76]. The transcription factors Clock and Bmal1, which form heterodimers and bind to an E-box enhancer element, regulate gene transcription [77, 78]. Bmal1 and Clock activate the genes Per and Cry. Once a certain concentration of PER and CRY proteins accumulate, they form BMAL1–CLOCK complex, consequently inhibiting gene transcription (**Figure 2**) [79, 80].

Clock–Bmal1 is not simply a passive consequence of negative feedback protein but rather induces proactive regulation [81]. As the core component of molecular clock, the Clock–Bmal1 complex controls numerous clock genes [82]. This complex may activate as well as repress transcription, and the switch depends on the interaction of Clock–Bmal1 with Cry [83]. The Clock–Bmal1-dependent recruitment of HATs promotes the periodic disruption of Clock–Bmal1 [84]. Clock–Bmal1 as a signaling molecule resets the clock through the Ca^{2+}-dependent protein kinase C pathway [85, 86]. The cAMP response element-binding protein activates the Clock–Bmal1 complex that rapidly resets phase and mediates the acute transactivation of Clock–Bmal1, consequently inducing immediate-early Per1 transcription [87]. Clock–Bmal1

DNA binding promotes rhythmic chromatin opening and remodeling. It mediates the rhythmic transcription factors binding to Clock–Bmal1 and the transcriptional output, suggesting that Clock–Bmal1 drives rhythmic gene expression and biological functions [88].

3.4. Effects of PER and CRY on the aging process

The Per and Cry genes can combine with the E-box domain promoters using Clock and Bmal1, thus driving the transcription of messenger RNA [79, 80]. Per and Cry genes play a negative transcriptional feedback loop in mouse [89]. When PER and CRY proteins reach adequately high levels, they form dimer feedback to the nucleus. The Clock–Bmal1 complex is then binded to turn off transcription [4]. Regulatory kinases Case in Kinase I epsilon (CKIε) of rodents phosphorylates PER and degrades it to feed back to the cell nucleus [90, 91]. CKIε masks the mPER1 nuclear localization signal, and mPer2 causes mPer1–mPer2 heterodimer formation in the cytoplasm. Phosphorylation-dependent cytoplasmic retention may be the reason for CKIε regulating the mammalian circadian rhythm [91]. In aged animals, Per1 transcription is induced by light and reduced with a significantly longer delay to resynchronization [92], whereas in young animals, the disruption of the Per genes results in insensitivity to light [89, 93].

Advancing age reduces retinal sensitivity, which causes various age-related diseases. In elderly people, homeostatic sleep is association with the circadian clock gene Per3 in coding regions. The Per3 gene associates with a phase advance in the melatonin profile; therefore, elderly people experience more nocturnal wakefulness [5]. In situ hybridization for Per2 mRNA revealed that the age-related decrease in the diurnal rhythm amplitude in the hippocampus may aggravate cognitive deficits [94]. Pattern differences in clock gene expression can be associated with a depressive state. Under abnormal light–dark conditions, Per1 and Per2 genes may result in a depressive state [95]. The expression of rPer1, rPer2, or rCry1 mRNA is similar in both young and old SCN; however, when stimulated by light, aging reduces the gene expression [89]. A decreased Per gene expression suggests an impaired clock regulatory network and stress defense pathways may accelerate aging [96].

3.5. Effects of the SIRT1 gene on the aging process

Sirtuins belong to the silent information regulator (SIR)2 family of proteins [97, 98]. SIR2 and its orthologs regulate senescence in yeast, worms, and flies [99–101]. SIR2 retards senescence and extends the lifespan of diverse species through caloric restriction [101, 102]. Sirtuins are nicotinamide adenine dinucleotide (NAD^+)-dependent deacylases, which promote cell survival by suppressing apoptosis or senescence [103]. Sirtuins play key roles in expediting the resistance by increasing antioxidant pathways and facilitating DNA damage repair [104]. Seven mammalian sirtuins exist, and SIRT1 is one of the most crucial mammalian SIR2 orthologs [98]. SIRT1 is involved in cellular metabolism and circadian core clockwork machinery in biological systems [105]. The direct deacetylation activity and NAD^+ salvage pathway were found to correlate with SIRT1 in the circadian rhythm system [106]. In addition, SIRT1 regulates the Clock–Bmal1 complex, and deacetylates and degrades Per2 [79]. The SIRT1 activity contributes to disturbances in the acetylation of H3 and Bmal1 and transduces cellular metabolic signals [105]. Moreover, SIRT1 has multiple downstream targets, including p53, Ku70, nuclear factor-kappaB, forkhead box O factors, peroxisome proliferator-activated receptor (PPAR) gamma coactivator 1-alpha (PCG-1α), PPARγ [98].

The central pacemaker is activated by SIRT1 to maintain robust circadian, and its decaying may accelerate aging [107]. SIRT1 can produce moderate changes in the intrinsic circadian period and is associated with age-related decline in the central clock. Some studies have reported a possible association between aging, sirtuins, and clock genes. SIRT1 activates the transcription of Bmal1 through PGC-1α to increase the amplitude of expression of BMAL1 and other proteins to control circadian rhythms in the SCN [108]. Recent studies have suggested that caloric restriction is a nongenetic manipulation that extends the lifespan; it is beneficial because SIRT1 has led to the search for sirtuin activators [109]. SIRT1 avoids mice getting diet-induced obesity by deacetylating and activating PGC-1α in the skeletal muscles [110]. In addition, the activity of the adipogenic nuclear receptor PPARγ is repressed by SIRT1 activation, thus reducing fat accumulation and adipocyte differentiation [98]. Moreover, SIRT1 mediates the lifespan extension through caloric restriction, affecting metabolism and lifespan in humans.

3.6. Effects of the ROR gene on the aging process

RORs are considered a core clock machinery because they regulate the cyclic expression of Bmal1 and Clock, thus providing an essential link between the positive and negative loops of the circadian clock [111]. RORs can be classified into three types: RORα, RORβ, and RORγ. RORα is the first member of the ROR subfamily and resembles the retinoic acid receptors and RXRs [112]. Both RORα and RORβ are required for the maturation of photoreceptors in the retina, and RORγ affects the development of several secondary lymphoid tissues [113].

RORα, an orphan nuclear receptor, plays a crucial role in integrating the circadian clock and regulating the cardiovascular function. Four RORα isoforms exist in humans, namely RORα1–4, whereas only two isoforms α1 and α4 are present in mouse [114]. These isoforms participate in the different physiological processes and exhibit a distinct pattern of tissue-specific expression. For example, the expression of RORα1 and RORα4 was significantly higher in mouse cerebellum than in other tissues, whereas RORα4 is predominantly expressed in liver tissues [115]. RORα and REV–ERBα compete for the binding of their shared DNA-binding elements in the Bmal1 promoter (**Figure 2**) [116, 117]. RORα displays rhythmic expression patterns during the circadian cycle in some tissues. RORα expression shows a weak circadian oscillation in the liver, kidneys, retina, and lungs [114, 118, 119]. Moreover, RORα promotes Bmal1 transcription [116] through two RORα autonomous response elements [118]. RORα1 enhances the circadian amplitude of Bmal1 mRNA expression and regulates the downstream clock genes after serum shock [118]. In addition, the reduced expression of RORα is closely associated with aging in genetic hypertensive rats [120]. The enhancement of the RORα expression was shown to antiaging in human endothelial cells by facilitating Bmal1 transcription, [121]. The deficiency of RORα causes cerebellar hypoplasia and affects Purkinje cell survival and differentiation in aging [122]. RORα has been shown to restraint age-related degenerative, including muscular atrophy, immune deficiencies, osteoporosis, atherosclerosis, and inflammation [123,

124]. RORα plays a neuroprotective role during development and provides protection against this injury [124].

3.7. Effects of the REV–ERBα gene on the aging process

REV–ERB nuclear receptors are considered to be essential core clock components and serve as pivotal regulators of rhythmic metabolism [125]. REV–ERB has α and β isoforms, which coexpression in adipose tissues and the liver and brain [126, 127]. REV–ERBα, an orphan nuclear receptor, negatively regulates the activity of the Clock–Bmal1 complex. Its transcription is controlled through Per and Cry transcription [128]. REV–ERBα competes with activators of the ROR family of nuclear receptors for binding to specific ROR-responsive elements to ensure the rhythmic transcription of Bmal1 and Clock [118, 129]. The development of metabolic disorders indicates disrupted circadian rhythms [111]. REV–ERBA is associated with circadian rhythms and metabolism and is pivotal in regulating the core mammalian molecular clock (**Figure 2**). Furthermore, REV–ERBα controls the transcription of metabolic pathways while serving as a crucial output regulator.

Age is the essential risk factor for metabolic syndrome. REV–ERBα connects the core clock and numerous physiological processes. The deficiency of REV–ERBα results in asynchronous circadian rhythms, with a tendency for diet-induced obesity, impaired glucose, and lipid utilization leading to an increased risk of diabetes [130]. Evidence suggests that REV–ERB has opened new avenues for treating metabolic syndrome by affecting the circadian rhythm and metabolism [111]: for example, targeting REV–ERBα as a critical component of the peripheral clock to treat bipolar disorder by affecting glycogen synthase kinase 3 [131]. REV–ERB agonists can reduce dyslipidemia, hyperglycemia syndromes, and obesity [130, 132].

4. Drug discovery

New biological targets are being developed for discovering novel drugs. People can identify with aging, thus antiaging drugs constitute a lucrative market. Medical therapy contributes in delaying the aging process in humans. Researchers focus not only on the compounds having a validated target but also on herbs used as antiaging products in traditional medicine. Some drugs used to treat chronic diseases can be examined; these diseases are associated with senescence, such as cardiovascular diseases, type 2 diabetes mellitus, and cancer. Some studies on the compounds have been conducted, whereas studies on herbs are necessary. Many lead compounds and approved drugs are derived from herbs. In China, traditional Chinese medicine (TCM) has been investigated in large-scale clinical trials, with extensive research on aging concerns. With the development of longevity drugs, Chinese herbs have been demonstrated to retard aging, such as *Polygonum multiflorum*, Ginseng. Meanwhile, TCM is gradually attracting worldwide attention.

4.1. Compounds as antiaging drugs

4.1.1. Rapamycin

Rapamycin, used as an immunosuppressive drug, has been recently considered for antiaging treatments. Rapamycin retards multiple aspects of aging, including extending the lifespan and slowing aging in mice [133]. Rapamycin evidences an association between metabolism and longevity by controlling the target of rapamycin kinases to regulate cell growth and proliferation through mitogenic signals [134]. In addition, rapamycin extends mouse lifespan principally by inhibiting many aspects of cancer development [135]. Rapamycin appears to retard the effects of age on the liver, endometrium [133], and bone marrow [136]. Rapamycin was shown to reduce the effects of aging in mice [137]; it can retard clinically relevant β-amyloid and tau accumulation in aged CNS tissues [138].

4.1.2. Resveratrol

Resveratrol, a natural phenol, retards aging by selective SIRT1 activation. Resveratrol as an established antioxidant has multiple beneficial activities and delays the onset of age-associated diseases. Resveratrol can reduce the expression of SIRT1 by using an acetylated substrate and NAD^+ [109]. In yeast, resveratrol extends the lifespan by upregulating Sir2 or increasing DNA stability [99]. Resveratrol has antioxidant, antiaging, and antiangiogenic properties. Furthermore, resveratrol plays a dual role on the vasculature; it maintains vascular fitness through its anti-inflammatory and anticoagulant activities, whereas it inhibits angiogenesis to suppress tumor growth [139].

4.2. Herbs as antiaging drugs

4.2.1. *Polygonum multiflorumygonum multiflorum*

Polygonum multiflorum, a crucial TCM, is extensively used for health maintenance and disease treatment, particularly as an antiaging drug in China. An active component extracted from the roots of P. *multiflorum* Thunb is called 2,3,5,4'-tetrahydroxystilbene-2-O-β-d-glucoside (THSG). THSG, the major bioactive compound of *P. multiflorum*, has antioxidant [140], anti-inflammatory [141], and endothelial-protective activities [142]. Our previous study revealed that THSG prevents vascular senescence by increasing eNOS expression and SIRT1 activity and reducing the acetylation of p53 at the K373 site [143]. In another study, we indicated that THSG extends the lifespan by promoting the expression of the longevity gene Klotho [144]. The antioxidant capacity of THSG is similar to resveratrol or even stronger. Moreover, THSG possesses a potent antioxidant capacity and extends the lifetime of the nematode *Caenorhabditis elegans* [145]. THSG is a potent antiaging drug and has potential as a pharmaceutical antiaging drug.

4.2.2. Ginseng

Ginseng is a highly valued herb in Asia and is recorded in Chinese Pharmacopoeia. The major active components of ginseng are ginsenosides. The beneficial effects of ginseng have been investigated; ginseng and its constituents have antianemic, antiaging, antioxidant, antineoplastic, and anti-stress activities. Rg1 and Rb1 improve the spatial learning ability by increasing the hippocampal synaptic density [109, 110]. Ginseng could play a crucial role in enhancing the defense system during the aging process. The mechanisms of ginsenosides warrant further investigation.

5. Conclusion

Considerable progress has been made to unravel the association between the circadian clock and aging. The role of circadian clocks in governing many other physiological systems has been reported; however, sufficient data are lacking. The circadian clock represents a nearly ubiquitous aspect of cellular regulation and molecular regulatory process, which exerts effects on organismal behavior. The researches on circadian clock genes regulation in aging have emerged recently, making the issue become attractive and outstanding.

The association between the circadian clock genes and aging might affect age-related diseases. The circadian clock is altered in normal aging, resulting in a decreased amplitude of rhythms in daily life, subsequently posing difficulties for humans to adjust to temporal changes. The study has major implications in determining why circadian rhythms diminish during aging and whether this decline could be reversed to tissue homeostasis and age-related diseases. However, additional studies are required to comprehensively understand the circadian clock effects on aging and obtain the target drug for extending the lifespan. Circadian genes must be extensively studied, including their different signaling pathways that are unknown, particularly the association between circadian genes and diseases. Focus on the effects of gene expression, translation, and signaling alterations on the biological clock would increase our knowledge regarding individualized treatment program and drug discovery.

Till date, studies have revealed several circadian clock genes that are crucial in regulating the lifespan. The manipulation of circadian clock genes would largely benefit the study of aging. This study not only explains circadian rhythm affects aging but also presents drugs for determining the therapeutic potential of targeting the circadian clock in diseases.

Author details

Yufeng Li, Yanqi Dang, Shuang Ling and Jin-Wen Xu*

*Address all correspondence to: jinwen.xu88@gmail.com

Murad Research Institute for Modernized Chinese Medicine, Shanghai University of Traditional Chinese Medicine, Shanghai, China

References

[1] Schibler U, Ripperger J, Brown SA. Peripheral circadian oscillators in mammals: time and food. Journal of Biological Rhythms. 2003;18:250–260. doi: 10.1177/0748730403253381.

[2] Yu EA, Weaver DR. Disrupting the circadian clock: gene-specific effects on aging, cancer, and other phenotypes. Aging (Albany NY). 2011;3:479–493. doi:10.18632/aging. 100323.

[3] Yuko M, Hideaki N, Katsuyuki M, Yoshiyuki S, Masao I, Teruhiko K, Yuchi N, Yasushi S, Koji N. Shift work and the risk of diabetes mellitus among Japanese male factory workers. Scandinavian Journal of Work Environment & Health. 2005;31:179–183. doi: 10.5271/sjweh.867.

[4] Gibson EM, Williams WP, 3rd, Kriegsfeld LJ. Aging in the circadian system: considerations for health, disease prevention and longevity. Experimental Gerontology. 2009;44:51–56. doi:10.1016/j.exger.2008.05.007.

[5] Viola AU, Chellappa SL, Archer SN, Pugin F, Gotz T, Dijk DJ, Cajochen C. Interindividual differences in circadian rhythmicity and sleep homeostasis in older people: effect of a PER3 polymorphism. Neurobiology of Aging. 2012;33:1010e17–27. doi: 10.1016/j.neurobiolaging.2011.10.024.

[6] Kunieda T, Minamino T, Katsuno T, Tateno K, Nishi J, Miyauchi H, Orimo M, Okada S, Komuro I. Cellular senescence impairs circadian expression of clock genes in vitro and in vivo. Circulation Research. 2006;98:532–539. doi:10.1161/01.RES. 0000204504.25798.a8.

[7] Takahashi JS, Hong HK, Ko CH, McDearmon EL. The genetics of mammalian circadian order and disorder: implications for physiology and disease. Nature Reviews Genetics. 2008;9:764–775. doi:10.1038/nrg2430.

[8] Fuhr L, Abreu M, Pett P, Relogio A. Circadian systems biology: when time matters. Computational and Structural Biotechnology Journal. 2015;13:417–426. doi:10.1016/ j.csbj.2015.07.001.

[9] Balsalobre A, Damiola F, Schibler U. A serum shock induces circadian gene expression in mammalian tissue culture cells. Cell. 1998;93:929–937. doi:10.1016/ S0092-8674(00)81199-X.

[10] Nagoshi E, Saini C, Bauer C, Laroche T, Naef F, Schibler U. Circadian gene expression in individual fibroblasts: cell-autonomous and self-sustained oscillators pass time to daughter cells. Cell. 2004;119:693–705. doi:10.1016/j.cell.2004.11.015.

[11] Mohawk JA, Green CB, Takahashi JS. Central and peripheral circadian clocks in mammals. Annual Review of Neuroscience. 2012;35:445–462. doi:10.1146/annurev-neuro-060909-153128.

[12] Reppert SM, Weaver DR. Molecular analysis of mammalian circadian rhythms. Annual Review of Physiology. 2001;63:647–676. doi:10.1146/annurev.physiol.63.1.647.

[13] Herzog ED. Neurons and networks in daily rhythms. Nature Reviews Neuroscience. 2007;8:790–802. doi:10.1038/nrn2215.

[14] Welsh DK, Logothetis DE, Meister M,., Reppert SM. Individual neurons dissociated from rat suprachiasmatic nucleus express independently phased circadian firing rhythms. Neuron. 1995;14:697–706. doi:10.1016/0896-6273(95)90214-7.

[15] Welsh DK, Yoo SH, Liu AC, Takahashi JS, Kay SA. Bioluminescence imaging of individual fibroblasts reveals persistent, independently phased circadian rhythms of clock gene expression. Current Biology. 2004;14:2289–2295. doi:10.1016/j.cub.2004.11.057.

[16] Welsh DK, Takahashi JS, Kay SA. Suprachiasmatic nucleus: cell autonomy and network properties. Annual Review of Physiology. 2010;72:551–577. doi:10.1146/annurev-physiol-021909-135919.

[17] Morin LP, Allen CN. The circadian visual system, 2005. Brain Research Reviews. 2006;51:1–60. doi:10.1016/j.brainresrev.2005.08.003.

[18] Aton SJ, Herzog ED. Come together, right…now: synchronization of rhythms in a mammalian circadian clock. Neuron. 2005;48:531–534. doi:10.1016/j.neuron.2005.11.001.

[19] Dibner C, Schibler U, Albrecht U. The mammalian circadian timing system: organization and coordination of central and peripheral clocks. Annual Review of Physiology. 2010;72:517–549. doi:10.1146/annurev-physiol-021909-135821.

[20] Richards J, Gumz ML. Advances in understanding the peripheral circadian clocks. Faseb Journal. 2012 September;26:3602–3613. doi:10.1096/fj.12-203554.

[21] Evans JA, Leise TL, Castanon-Cervantes O, Davidson AJ. Intrinsic regulation of spatiotemporal organization within the suprachiasmatic nucleus. PLoS One. 2011;6:e15869. doi:10.1371/journal.pone.0015869.

[22] Shun Y, Hiromi I, Takuya M, Ryusuke O, Kazuhiro Y, Masaki K, Hitoshi O. Synchronization of cellular clocks in the suprachiasmatic nucleus. Science. 2003;302:1408–14012. doi:10.1126/science.1089287.

[23] Inagaki N, Honma S, Ono D, Tanahashi Y, Honma K. Separate oscillating cell groups in mouse suprachiasmatic nucleus couple photoperiodically to the onset and end of daily activity. Proceedings of the National Academy of Sciences of the United States of America. 2007;104:7664–7669. doi:10.1073/pnas.0607713104.

[24] Yagita K, Tamanini F, Horst GTVD, Van Der, Okamura H. Molecular mechanisms of the biological clock in cultured fibroblasts. Science. 2001;292:278–281. doi:10.1126/science.1059542.

[25] Yamazaki S, Numano R, Abe M, Hida A, Takahashi R, Ueda M, Block GD, Sakaki Y, Menaker M, Tei H. Resetting central and peripheral circadian oscillators in transgenic rats. Science. 2000;288:682–685. doi:10.1126/science.288.5466.682.

[26] Gachon F, Olela FF, Schaad O, Descombes P, Schibler U. The circadian PAR-domain basic leucine zipper transcription factors DBP, TEF, and HLF modulate basal and inducible xenobiotic detoxification. Cell Metabolism. 2006;4:25–36. doi:10.1016/j.cmet.2006.04.015.

[27] Kornmann B, Schaad O, Reinke H, Saini C, Schibler U. Regulation of circadian gene expression in liver by systemic signals and hepatocyte oscillators. Cold Spring Harbor Symposia on Quantitative Biology. 2007;72:319–330. doi:10.1101/sqb.2007.72.041.

[28] Stratmann M, Schibler U. Properties, entrainment, and physiological functions of mammalian peripheral oscillators. Journal of Biological Rhythms. 2006;21:494–506. doi:10.1177/0748730406293889.

[29] Damiola F, Le Minh N, Preitner N, Kornmann B, Fleury-Olela F, Schibler U. Restricted feeding uncouples circadian oscillators in peripheral tissues from the central pacemaker in the suprachiasmatic nucleus. Genes & Development. 2001;14:2950–2961. doi:10.1101/gad.183500.

[30] Buijs R, Hermes MHLJ, Kalsbeek A. The suprachiasmatic nucleus—paraventricular nucleus interactions: a bridge to the neuroendocrine and autonomic nervous system. Progress in Brain Research. 1998;119:365–382. doi:10.1016/s0079-6123(08)61581-2.

[31] Albrecht U. Timing to perfection: the biology of central and peripheral circadian clocks. Neuron. 2012;74:246–260. doi:10.1016/j.neuron.2012.04.006.

[32] Relogio A, Westermark PO, Wallach T, Schellenberg K, Kramer A, Herzel H. Tuning the mammalian circadian clock: robust synergy of two loops. Plos Computational Biology. 2011;7:e1002309. doi:10.1371/journal.pcbi.1002309.

[33] Oishi K. Plasminogen activator inhibitor-1 and the circadian clock in metabolic disorders. Clinical and Experimental Hypertension. 2009;31:208–219. doi:10.1080/10641960902822468.

[34] Duez H, Staels B. The nuclear receptors Rev-erbs and RORs integrate circadian rhythms and metabolism. Diabetes & Vascular Disease Research. 2008;5:82–88. doi:10.3132/dvdr.2008.0014.

[35] Maury E, Ramsey KM, Bass J. Circadian rhythms and metabolic syndrome: from experimental genetics to human disease. Circulation Research. 2010;106:447–462. doi:10.1161/CIRCRESAHA.109.208355.

[36] Knutson KL, Spiegel K, Penev P, Van Cauter E. The metabolic consequences of sleep deprivation. Sleep Medicine Reviews. 2007;11:163–178. doi:10.1016/j.smrv.2007.01.002.

[37] Philippe J, Dibner C. Thyroid circadian timing: roles in physiology and thyroid malignancies. Journal of Biological Rhythms. 2015;30:76–83. doi: 10.1177/0748730414557634.

[38] Wood S, Loudon A. Clocks for all seasons: unwinding the roles and mechanisms of circadian and interval timers in the hypothalamus and pituitary. Journal of Endocrinology. 2014;222:R39–59. doi:10.1530/JOE-14-0141.

[39] Bailey M, Silver R. Sex differences in circadian timing systems: implications for disease. Frontiers in Neuroendocrinology. 2014;35:111–139. doi:10.1016/j.yfrne.2013.11.003.

[40] Tomoshige K. Circadian rhythms of glucocorticoid hormone actions in target tissues: potential clinical implications. Science Signaling. 2012;5:3949–50. doi:10.1126/scisignal.2003333.

[41] Sellix MT. Clocks underneath: the role of peripheral clocks in the timing of female reproductive physiology. Front in Endocrinology (Lausanne). 2013;4:91. doi:10.3389/fendo.2013.00091.

[42] Williams WP, 3rd, Kriegsfeld LJ. Circadian control of neuroendocrine circuits regulating female reproductive function. Front in Endocrinology (Lausanne). 2012;3:60. doi: 10.3389/fendo.2012.00060.

[43] Valenzuela FJ, Vera J, Venegas C, Pino F, Lagunas C. Circadian system and melatonin hormone: risk factors for complications during pregnancy. International Journal of Gynecology & Obstetrics. 2015;2015:1–10. doi:10.1155/2015/825802.

[44] Seron-Ferre M, Valenzuela GJ, Torres-Farfan C. Circadian clocks during embryonic and fetal development. Birth Defects Research Part C – Embryo Today: Reviews. 2007;81:204–214. doi:10.1002/bdrc.20101.

[45] Torres-Farfan C, Rocco V, Monsó C, Valenzuela FJ, Campino C, Germain A, Torrealba F, Valenzuela GJ, Seron-Ferre M. Maternal melatonin effects on clock gene expression in a nonhuman primate fetus. Endocrinology. 2006;147:4618–4626. doi:10.1210/en.2006-0628.

[46] Bollinger T, Bollinger A, Oster H, Solbach W. Sleep, immunity, and circadian clocks: a mechanistic model. Gerontology. 2010;56:574–580. doi:10.1159/000281827.

[47] Kyriacou CP, Hastings MH. Circadian clocks: genes, sleep, and cognition. Trends in Cognitive Sciences. 2010;14:259–267. doi:10.1016/j.tics.2010.03.007.

[48] Kawakami F, Okamura H, Tamada Y, Maebayashi Y, Fukui K, Ibata Y. Loss of day-night differences in VIP mRNA levels in the suprachiasmatic nucleus of aged rats. Neuroscience Letters. 1997;222:99–102. doi:10.1016/S0304-3940(97)13355-9.

[49] Satinoff E, Li H, Tcheng TK, Liu C, McArthur AJ, Medanic M, Gillette MU. Do the suprachiasmatic nuclei oscillate in old rats as they do in young ones? American Journal of Physiology. 1993;265:R1216-1222. doi:10.1109/ICNSC.2005.1461293.

[50] Cai A, Scarbrough K, Hinkle DA, Wise PM. Fetal grafts containing suprachiasmatic nuclei restore the diurnal rhythm of CRH and POMC mRNA in aging rats. American Journal of Physiology. 1997;273(5 Pt 2):R1764–1770.

[51] Satchidananda P, Hogenesch JB, Kay SA. Circadian rhythms from flies to human. Nature. 2002;417:329–335. doi:10.1038/417329a.

[52] Khapre RV, Kondratova AA, Susova O, Kondratov RV. Circadian clock protein BMAL1 regulates cellular senescence in vivo. Cell Cycle. 2011;10:4162–4169. doi:10.4161/cc.10.23.18381.

[53] Kondratov RV, Kondratova AA, Gorbacheva VY, Vykhovanets OV, Antoch MP. Early aging and age-related pathologies in mice deficient in BMAL1, the core componentof the circadian clock. Genes & Development. 2006;20:1868–1873. doi:10.4161/cc.10.23.18381.

[54] Somanath PR, Podrez EA, Chen J, Ma Y, Marchant K, Antoch M, Byzova TV. Deficiency in core circadian protein Bmal1 is associated with a prothrombotic and vascular phenotype. Journal of Cellular Physiology. 2011;226:132–140. doi:10.1002/jcp.22314.

[55] Young ME, Brewer RA, Peliciari-Garcia RA, Collins HE, He L, Birky TL, Peden BW, Thompson EG, Ammons BJ, Bray MS, Chatham JC, Wende AR, Yang Q, Chow CW, Martino TA, Gamble KL. Cardiomyocyte-specific BMAL1 plays critical roles in metabolism, signaling, and maintenance of contractile function of the heart. Journal of Biological Rhythms. 2014;29:257–276. doi:10.1002/jcp.22314.

[56] Razorenova OV. Brain and muscle ARNT-like protein BMAL1 regulates ROS homeostasis and senescence: a possible link to hypoxia-inducible factor-mediated pathway. Cell Cycle. 2012;11:213–214. doi:10.4161/cc.11.2.18786.

[57] Khapre RV, Kondratova AA, Patel S, Dubrovsky Y, Wrobel M, Antoch MP, Kondratov RV. BMAL1-dependent regulation of the mTOR signaling pathway delays aging. Aging (Albany NY). 2014;6:48–57. doi:10.18632/aging.100633.

[58] Lefta M, Campbell KS, Feng HZ, Jin JP, Esser KA. Development of dilated cardiomyopathy in Bmal1-deficient mice. American Journal of Physiology-heart and Circulatory Physiology. 2012;303:H475–485. doi:10.1152/ajpheart.00238.2012.

[59] Hemmeryckx B, Van Hove CE, Fransen P, Emmerechts J, Kauskot A, Bult H, Lijnen HR, Hoylaerts MF. Progression of the prothrombotic state in aging Bmal1-deficient mice. Arteriosclerosis Thrombosis and Vascular Biology. 2011;31:2552–2559. doi:10.1152/ajpheart.00238.2012.

[60] Dubrovsky YV, Samsa WE, Kondratov RV. Deficiency of circadian protein CLOCK reduces lifespan and increases age-related cataract development in mice. Aging (Albany NY). 2010;2:936–944. doi:10.18632/aging.100241.

[61] Antoch MP, Song EJ, Chang AM, Vitaterna MH, Zhao Y, Wilsbacher LD, Sangoram AM, King DP, Pinto LH, Takahashi JS. Functional identification of the mouse circadian

clock gene by transgenic BAC rescue. Cell. 1997;89:655–667. doi:10.1016/S0092-8674(00)80246-9.

[62] King DP, Zhao Y, Sangoram AM, Wilsbacher LD, Tanaka M, Antoch MP, Steeves TD, Vitaterna MH, Kornhauser JM, Lowrey PL. Positional cloning of the mouse circadian clock gene. Cell. 1997;89:641–653. doi:10.1016/S0092-8674(00)80245-7.

[63] Debruyne JP, Noton E, Lambert CM, Maywood ES, Weaver DR, Reppert SM. A clock shock: mouse CLOCK is not required for circadian oscillator function. Neuron. 2006;50:465–477. doi:10.1016/j.neuron.2006.03.041.

[64] Lee C, Etchegaray J-P, Cagampang FRA, Loudon ASI, Reppert SM. Posttranslational mechanisms regulate the mammalian circadian clock. Cell. 2001;107:855–867. doi:10.1016/s0092-8674(01)00610-9.

[65] DeBruyne JP, Weaver DR, Reppert SM. CLOCK and NPAS2 have overlapping roles in the suprachiasmatic circadian clock. Nature Neuroscience. 2007;10:543–545. doi:10.1038/nn1884.

[66] Kolker DE, Vitaterna MH, Fruechte EM, Takahashi JS, Turek FW. Effects of age on circadian rhythms are similar in wild-type and heterozygous Clock mutant mice. Neurobiology of Aging. 2004;25:517–523. doi:10.1016/j.neurobiolaging.2003.06.007.

[67] Jin X, Shearman LP, Weaver DR, Zylka MJ, Vries GJ, De, Reppert SM. A molecular mechanism regulating rhythmic output from the suprachiasmatic circadian clock. Cell. 1999;96:57–68. doi:10.1016/S0092-8674(00)80959-9.

[68] Darlington TK. Closing the circadian loop: CLOCK-induced transcription of Its own inhibitors per and tim. Science. 1998;280:1599–1603. doi:10.1126/science.280.5369.1599.

[69] Kolker DE, Fukuyama H, Huang DS, Takahashi JS, Horton TH, Turek FW. Aging alters circadian and light-induced expression of clock genes in golden hamsters. Journal of Biological Rhythms. 2003;18:159–169. doi:10.1177/0748730403251802.

[70] Debruyne JP, Weaver DR, Reppert SM. Peripheral circadian oscillators require CLOCK. Current Biology. 2007;17:R538–539. doi:10.1016/j.cub.2007.05.067.

[71] Gekakis N. Role of the CLOCK protein in the mammalian circadian mechanism. Science. 1998;280:1564–1569. doi:10.1126/science.280.5369.1564.

[72] Duong HA, Robles MS, Knutti D, Weitz CJ. A molecular mechanism for circadian clock negative feedback. Science. 2011;332:1436–1439. doi:10.1126/science.1196766.

[73] Padmanabhan K, Robles MS, Westerling T, Weitz CJ. Feedback regulation of transcriptional termination by the mammalian circadian clock PERIOD complex. Science. 2012;337:599–602. doi:10.1126/science.1221592.

[74] Doi M, Hirayama J, Sassone-Corsi P. Circadian regulator CLOCK is a histone acetyltransferase. Cell. 2006;125:497–508. doi:10.1016/j.cell.2006.03.033.

[75] Katada S, Sassone-Corsi P. The histone methyltransferase MLL1 permits the oscillation of circadian gene expression. Nature Structural & Molecular Biology. 2010;17:1414–1421. doi:10.1038/nsmb.1961.

[76] DiTacchio L, Le HD, Vollmers C, Hatori M, Witcher M, Secombe J, Panda S. Histone lysine demethylase JARID1a activates CLOCK-BMAL1 and influences the circadian clock. Science. 2011;333:1881–1185. doi:10.1126/science.1206022.

[77] Rudic RD, McNamara P, Curtis AM, Boston RC, Panda S, Hogenesch JB, Fitzgerald GA. BMAL1 and CLOCK, two essential components of the circadian clock, are involved in glucose homeostasis. PLoS Biology. 2004;2:1893–1899. doi:10.1371/journal.pbio.0020377.

[78] Huang N, Chelliah Y, Shan Y, Taylor CA, Yoo SH, Partch C, Green CB, Zhang H, Takahashi JS. Crystal structure of the heterodimeric CLOCK:BMAL1 transcriptional activator complex. Science. 2012;337:189–194. doi:10.1126/science.1222804.

[79] Asher G, Gatfield D, Stratmann M, Reinke H, Dibner C, Kreppel F, Mostoslavsky R, Alt FW, Schibler U. SIRT1 regulates circadian clock gene expression through PER2 deacetylation. Cell. 2008;134:317–328. doi:10.1016/j.cell.2008.06.050.

[80] Kume K, Zylka MJ, Sriram S, Shearman LP, Weaver DR, Jin X, Maywood ES, Hastings MH, Reppert SM. mCRY1 and mCRY2 are essential components of the negative limb of the circadian clock feedback loop. Cell. 1999;98:193–205. doi:10.1016/s0092-8674(00)81014-4.

[81] Koike N, Yoo SH, Huang HC, Kumar V, Lee C, Kim TK, Takahashi JS. Transcriptional architecture and chromatin landscape of the core circadian clock in mammals. Science. 2012;338:349–354. doi:10.1126/science.1226339.

[82] Reppert SM, Weaver DR. Coordination of circadian timing in mammals. Nature. 2002;418:935–941. doi:10.1038/nature00965.

[83] Kondratov RV, Shamanna RK, Kondratova AA, Gorbacheva VY, Antoch MP. Dual role of the CLOCK/BMAL1 circadian complex in transcriptional regulation. Faseb Journal. 2006;20:530–532. doi:10.1096/fj.05-5321fje.

[84] Jean-Pierre E, Choogon L, Wade PA, Reppert SM. Rhythmic histone acetylation underlies transcription in the mammalian circadian clock. Nature. 2003;421:177–182. doi:10.1038/nature01314.

[85] Jung H, Choe Y, Kim H, Park N, Son GH, Khang I, Kim K. Involvement of CLOCK.BMAL1 heterodimer in serum-responsive mPer1 induction. Neuroreport. 2003;14:15–19. doi:10.1097/01.wnr.0000050715.17082.d2.

[86] Shim HS, Kim H, Lee J, Son GH, Cho S, Oh TH, Kang SH, Seen DS, Lee KH, Kim K. Rapid activation of CLOCK by Ca^{2+}-dependent protein kinase C mediates resetting of the mammalian circadian clock. EMBO Reports. 2007;8:366–371. doi:10.1038/sj.embor.7400920.

[87] Lee Y, Lee J, Kwon I, Nakajima Y, Ohmiya Y, Son GH, Lee KH, Kim K. Coactivation of the CLOCK-BMAL1 complex by CBP mediates resetting of the circadian clock. Journal of Cell Science. 2010;123:3547–3557. doi:10.1242/jcs.070300.

[88] Menet JS, Pescatore S, Rosbash M. CLOCK:BMAL1 is a pioneer-like transcription factor. Genes & Development. 2014;28(1):8–13. doi:10.1101/gad.228536.113.

[89] Asai M, Yoshinobu Y, Kaneko S, Mori A, Nikaido T, Moriya T, Akiyama M, Shibata S. Circadian profile of Per gene mRNA expression in the suprachiasmatic nucleus, paraventricular nucleus, and pineal body of aged rats. Journal of Neuroscience Research. 2001;66:1133–1139. doi:10.1002/jnr.10010.abs.

[90] Lowrey PL, Shimomura K, Antoch MP, Yamazaki S, Zemenides PD, Ralph MR, Menaker M, Takahashi JS. Positional syntenic cloning and functional characterization of the mammalian circadian mutation tau. Science. 2000;288:483–492. doi:10.1126/science.288.5465.483.

[91] Vielhaber E, Eide E, Rivers A, Gao ZH, Virshup DM. Nuclear entry of the circadian regulator mPER1 Is controlled by mammalian casein kinase I varepsilon. Molecular and Cellular Biology. 2000;20:4888–4899. doi:10.1128/mcb.20.13.4888-4899.2000.

[92] Davidson AJ, Yamazaki S, Arble DM, Menaker M, Block GD. Resetting of central and peripheral circadian oscillators in aged rats. Neurobiology of Aging. 2008;29:471–477. doi:10.1016/j.neurobiolaging.2006.10.018.

[93] Weinert H, Weinert D, Schurov I, Maywood ES, Hastings MH. Impaired expression of the mPer2 circadian clock gene in the suprachiasmatic nuclei of aging mice. Chronobiology International. 2001;18:559–565. doi:10.1081/CBI-100103976.

[94] Duncan MJ, Prochot JR, Cook DH, Tyler Smith J, Franklin KM. Influence of aging on Bmal1 and Per2 expression in extra-SCN oscillators in hamster brain. Brain Research. 2013;1491:44–53. doi:10.1016/j.brainres.2012.11.008.

[95] Moriya S, Tahara Y, Sasaki H, Ishigooka J, Shibata S. Housing under abnormal light–dark cycles attenuates day/night expression rhythms of the clock genes Per1, Per2, and Bmal1 in the amygdala and hippocampus of mice. Neuroscience Research. 2015;99:16–21. doi:10.1016/j.neures.2015.05.005.

[96] Krishnan N, Kretzschmar D, Rakshit K, Chow E, Giebultowicz JM. The circadian clock gene period extends healthspan in aging Drosophila melanogaster. Aging (Albany NY). 2009;1:937–948. doi:10.18632/aging.100103.

[97] Blander G, Guarente L. The Sir2 family of protein deacetylases. Annual Review of Biochemistry. 2004;73:417–35. doi:10.1146/annurev.biochem.73.011303.073651.

[98] Dali-Youcef N, Lagouge M, Froelich S, Koehl C, Schoonjans K, Auwerx J. Sirtuins: the 'magnificent seven', function, metabolism and longevity. Annals of Medicine. 2007;39:335–345. doi:10.1080/07853890701408194.

[99] Howitz KT, Bitterman KJ, Cohen HY, Lamming DW, Siva L, Wood JG, Zipkin RE, Phuong C, Anne K, Li-Li Z. Small molecule activators of sirtuins extend *Saccharomyces cerevisiae* lifespan. Nature. 2003;425:191–196. doi:10.1038/nature01960.

[100] Kaeberlein M, McVey M, Guarente L. The SIR2/3/4 complex and SIR2 alone promote longevity in *Saccharomyces cerevisiae* by two different mechanisms. Genes & Development. 1999;13:2570–2580. doi:10.1101/gad.13.19.2570.

[101] Rogina B, Helfand SL. Sir2 mediates longevity in the fly through a pathway related to calorie restriction. Proceedings of the National Academy of Sciences of the United States of America. 2004;101:15998–6003. doi:10.1073/pnas.0404184101.

[102] Lin SJ. Requirement of NAD and SIR2 for life-span extension by calorie restriction in *Saccharomyces cerevisiae*. Science. 2000;289:2126–2128. doi:10.1126/science.289.5487.2126.

[103] Jung-Hynes B, Ahmad N. SIRT1 controls circadian clock circuitry and promotes cell survival: a connection with age-related neoplasms. Faseb Journal. 2009;23:2803–2809. doi:10.1096/fj.09-129148.

[104] Imai S, Guarente L. NAD^+ and sirtuins in aging and disease. Trends in Cell Biology. 2014;24:464–471. doi:10.1016/j.tcb.2014.04.002.

[105] Nakahata Y, Kaluzova M, Grimaldi B, Sahar S, Hirayama J, Chen D, Guarente LP, Sassone-Corsi P. The NAD^+-dependent deacetylase SIRT1 modulates CLOCK-mediated chromatin remodeling and circadian control. Cell. 2008;134:329–340. doi:10.1016/j.cell.2008.07.002.

[106] Jung-Hynes B, Reiter RJ, Ahmad N. Sirtuins, melatonin and circadian rhythms: building a bridge between aging and cancer. Journal of Pineal Research. 2010;48:9–19. doi:10.1111/j.1600-079X.2009.00729.x.

[107] Satoh A, Stein L, Imai S. The role of mammalian sirtuins in the regulation of metabolism, aging, and longevity. Handbook Experimental Pharmacology. 2011;206:125–162. doi:10.1007/978-3-642-21631-2_7.

[108] Chang HC, Guarente L. SIRT1 mediates central circadian control in the SCN by a mechanism that decays with aging. Cell. 2013;153:1448–1460. doi:10.1016/j.cell.2013.05.027.

[109] Ramis MR, Esteban S, Miralles A, Tan D-X, Reiter RJ. Caloric restriction, resveratrol and melatonin: role of SIRT1 and implications for aging and related-diseases. Mechanisms of Ageing and Development. 2015;146:28–41. doi:10.1016/j.mad.2015.03.008.

[110] Rodgers JT, Lerin C, Haas W, Gygi SP, Spiegelman BM, Puigserver P. Nutrient control of glucose homeostasis through a complex of PGC-1alpha and SIRT1. Nature. 2005;434:113–118. doi:10.1038/nature03354.

[111] Marciano DP, Chang MR, Corzo CA, Goswami D, Lam VQ, Pascal BD, Griffin PR. The therapeutic potential of nuclear receptor modulators for treatment of metabolic

disorders: PPARgamma, RORs, and Rev-erbs. Cell Metabolism. 2014;19:193–208. doi: 10.1016/j.cmet.2013.12.009.

[112] Giguère V, Tini M, Flock G, Ong E. Evans RM, Otulakowski G. Isoform-specific amino-terminal domains dictate DNA-binding properties of ROR alpha, a novel family of orphan hormone nuclear receptors. Genes & Development. 1994;8:538–553. doi: 10.1101/gad.8.5.538.

[113] Jetten AM. Retinoid-related orphan receptors (RORs): critical roles in development, immunity, circadian rhythm, and cellular metabolism. Nuclear Receptor Signaling. 2009;7:1–32. doi:10.1621/nrs.07003.

[114] Andre E, Conquet F, Steinmayr M, Stratton SC, Porciatti V, Becker-Andre M. Disruption of retinoid-related orphan receptor beta changes circadian behavior, causes retinal degeneration and leads to vacillans phenotype in mice. EMBO Journal. 1998;17:3867–3877. doi:10.1093/emboj/17.14.3867.

[115] Caroline C, Brigitte BJ, Jean-Louis D. Retinoic acid receptor-related orphan receptor (ROR) alpha4 is the predominant isoform of the nuclear receptor RORalpha in the liver and is up-regulated by hypoxia in HepG2 human hepatoma cells. Biochemical Journal. 2002;364:449–456. doi:10.1042/BJ20011558.

[116] Guillaumond F, Dardente H, Giguere V, Cermakian N. Differential control of Bmal1 circadian transcription by REV-ERB and ROR nuclear receptors. Journal of Biological Rhythms. 2005;20:391–403. doi:10.1177/0748730405277232.

[117] Sato TK, Panda S, Miraglia LJ, Reyes TM, Rudic RD, McNamara P, Naik KA, FitzGerald GA, Kay SA, Hogenesch JB. A functional genomics strategy reveals Rora as a component of the mammalian circadian clock. Neuron. 2004;43:527–537. doi:10.1016/j.neuron.2004.07.018.

[118] Akashi M, Takumi T. The orphan nuclear receptor RORalpha regulates circadian transcription of the mammalian core-clock Bmal1. Nature Structural & Molecular Biology. 2005;12:441–448. doi:10.1038/nsmb925.

[119] Kamphuis W, Cailotto C, Dijk F, Bergen A, Buijs RM. Circadian expression of clock genes and clock-controlled genes in the rat retina. Biochemical and Biophysical Research Communications. 2005;330:18–26. doi:10.1016/j.bbrc.2005.02.118.

[120] Miyazaki M, Schroder E, Edelmann SE, Hughes ME, Kornacker K, Balke CW, Esser KA. Age-associated disruption of molecular clock expression in skeletal muscle of the spontaneously hypertensive rat. PLoS One. 2011;6:e27168. doi:10.1371/journal.pone.0027168.

[121] Dang Y, Ling S, Ma J, Ni R, Xu JW. Bavachalcone enhances RORalpha expression, controls bmal1 circadian transcription, and depresses cellular senescence in human endothelial cells. Evidence-based Complementary and Alternative Medicine. 2015;2015:920431. doi:10.1155/2015/920431.

[122] Boukhtouche F, Doulazmi M, Frederic F, Dusart I, Brugg B, Mariani J. RORalpha, a pivotal nuclear receptor for Purkinje neuron survival and differentiation: from development to ageing. Cerebellum. 2006;5:97–104. doi:10.1080/14734220600750184.

[123] Jarvis CI, Staels B, Brugg B, Lemaigre-Dubreuil Y, Tedgui A, Mariani J. Age-related phenotypes in the staggerer mouse expand the RORalpha nuclear receptor's role beyond the cerebellum. Molecular and Cellular Endocrinology. 2002;186:1–5. doi: 10.1016/S0303-7207(01)00668-2.

[124] Boukhtouche F, Mariani J, Tedgui A. The "CholesteROR" protective pathway in the vascular system. Arteriosclerosis Thrombosis and Vascular Biology. 2004;24:637–43. doi:10.1161/01.ATV.0000119355.56036.de.

[125] Stratmann M, Schibler U. REV-ERBs: more than the sum of the individual parts. Cell Metabolism. 2012;15:791–793. doi:10.1161/01.ATV.0000119355.56036.de.

[126] Bonnelye E, Vanacker JM, Desbiens X, Begue A, Stehelin D, Laudet V. Rev-erb β, a new member of the nuclear receptor superfamily, is expressed in the nervous system during chicken development. Cell Growth & Differentation. 1995;5:1357–1365.

[127] Bugge A, Feng D, Everett LJ, Briggs ER, Mullican SE, Wang F, Jager J, Lazar MA. Rev-erbalpha and Rev-erbbeta coordinately protect the circadian clock and normal metabolic function. Genes & Development. 2012;26:657–667. doi:10.1101/gad.186858.112.

[128] Ripperger JA, Schibler U. Rhythmic CLOCK-BMAL1 binding to multiple E-box motifs drives circadian Dbp transcription and chromatin transitions. Nature Genetics. 2006;38:369–374. doi:10.1038/ng1738.

[129] Preitner N, Damiola F, Zakany J, Duboule D. The orphan nuclear receptor REV-ERBα controls circadian transcription within the positive limb of the mammalian circadian oscillator. Cell. 2002;110:251–260. doi:10.1016/S0092-8674(02)00825-5.

[130] Delezie J, Dumont S, Dardente H, Oudart H, Grechez-Cassiau A, Klosen P, Teboul M, Delaunay F, Pevet P, Challet E. The nuclear receptor REV-ERBalpha is required for the daily balance of carbohydrate and lipid metabolism. Faseb Journal. 2012;26:3321–3335. doi:10.1096/fj.12-208751.

[131] Lei Y, Jing W, Klein PS, Lazar MA. Nuclear receptor Rev-erbalpha is a critical lithium-sensitive component of the circadian clock. Science. 2006;311:1002–1005. doi:10.1126/science.1121613.

[132] Ramakrishnan SN, Lau P, Burke LJ, Muscat GE. Rev-erbbeta regulates the expression of genes involved in lipid absorption in skeletal muscle cells: evidence for cross-talk between orphan nuclear receptors and myokines. Journal of Biological Chemistry. 2005;280:8651–8659. doi:10.1074/jbc.M413949200.

[133] Wilkinson JE, Burmeister L, Brooks SV, Chan CC, Friedline S, Harrison DE, Hejtmancik JF, Nadon N, Strong R, Wood LK, Woodward MA, .Miller RA. Rapamycin slows aging in mice. Aging Cell. 2012;11:675–682. doi: 10.1111/j.1474-9726.2012.00832.x

[134] Vellai T, Takacs-Vellai K, Zhang Y, Kovacs AL, Orosz L, Muller F. Genetics: influence of TOR kinase on lifespan in *C. elegans*. Nature. 2003;426:620–620. doi:10.1038/426620a.

[135] Hidalgo M, Rowinsky EK. The rapamycin-sensitive signal transduction pathway as a target for cancer therapy. Oncogene. 2000;19:6680–6686. doi:10.1038/sj.onc.1204091.

[136] Chen C, Liu Y, Liu Y, Zheng P. mTOR regulation and therapeutic rejuvenation of aging hematopoietic stem cells. Science Signaling. 2009;2:ra75. doi:10.1126/scisignal.2000559.

[137] Blagosklonny MV. Aging and immortality: quasi-programmed senescence and its pharmacologic inhibition. Cell Cycle. 2014;5:2087–2102. doi:10.4161/cc.5.18.3288.

[138] Caccamo A, Majumder S, Richardson A, Strong R, Oddo S. Molecular interplay between mammalian target of rapamycin (mTOR), amyloid-beta, and Tau: effects on cognitive impairments. Journal of Biological Chemistry. 2010;285:13107–13120. doi: 10.1074/jbc.M110.100420.

[139] Kasiotis KM, Pratsinis H, Kletsas D, Haroutounian SA. Resveratrol and related stilbenes: their anti-aging and anti-angiogenic properties. Food and Chemical Toxicology. 2013;61:112–120. doi:10.1016/j.fct.2013.03.038.

[140] Jing Z, Shouzhu X, Fan S, Lun N, Xuanxuan Z, Siwang W. 2,3,5,4′-tetrahydroxystilbene-2-O-β-D-glucoside protects human umbilical vein endothelial cells against lysophosphatidylcholine-induced apoptosis by upregulating superoxide dismutase and glutathione peroxidase. IUBMB Life. 2014;66:711–722. doi:10.1002/iub.1321.

[141] Huang C, Wang Y, Wang J, Yao W, Chen X, Zhang W. TSG (2,3,4′,5-tetrahydroxystilbene 2-O-β-D-glucoside) suppresses induction of pro-inflammatory factors by attenuating the binding activity of nuclear factor-kB in microglia. Journal of Neuroinflammation. 2013;10:1–12. doi:10.1186/1742-2094-10-129.

[142] Zhang W, Xu XL, Wang YQ, Wang CH, Zhu WZ. Effects of 2,3,4′,5-tetrahydroxystilbene 2-O-β-D-glucoside on vascular endothelial dysfunction in atherogenic-diet rats. Planta Medica. 2009;75:1209–1214. doi:10.1055/s-0029-1185540.

[143] Han X, Ling S, Gan W, Sun L, Duan J, Xu JW. 2,3,5,4′-tetrahydroxystilbene-2-O-β-d-glucoside ameliorates vascular senescence and improves blood flow involving a mechanism of p53 deacetylation. Atherosclerosis. 2012;225:76–82. doi:10.1016/j.atherosclerosis.2012.08.011.

[144] Ling S,Duan J,NI R. Xu JW. 2,3,5,4′-Tetrahydroxystilbene-2-O-β-D-glucoside promotes longevity gene klotho expression. Oxidative Medicine and Cellular Longevity. (in press).

[145] Buchter C, Zhao L, Havermann S, Honnen S, Fritz G, Proksch P, Watjen W. TSG (2,3,5,4′-tetrahydroxystilbene-2-O-beta-D-glucoside) from the Chinese Herb *Polygonum multiflorum* increases life span and stress resistance of *Caenorhabditis elegans*. Oxidative Medicine and Cellular Longevity. 2015;2015:124357. doi: 10.1155/2015/124357.

Chapter 3

Ion Channels in Aging and Aging-Related Diseases

Vidhya Rao, Simon Kaja and Saverio Gentile

Additional information is available at the end of the chapter

http://dx.doi.org/10.5772/63951

Abstract

Aging in humans is the decline over function of time of biological processes that include the capacity to grow, to reproduce, to interact, and to adapt, resulting in progressive organ malfunctions, illnesses, and ultimately death. As the average life expectancy is estimated to be above 60 years for about 25% of the world's population by 2050, understanding the causes of and designing treatments for aging-related disease is a compelling priority. Although every organ and tissue undergoes the process of aging, it appears that only few pathogeneses are typically detected with high frequency in elderly individuals. These include cardiovascular disease, neurodegeneration, vision loss, and cancer. Therefore, aging could be measured by monitoring the occurrence and progression of these diseases. However, each of these medical conditions alone is not a good marker for aging as elder patients present comorbid chronic conditions. In addition, treatment of one disease does not significantly prolong life expectancy. Therefore, it appears that a possible antiaging therapeutic strategy should consider simultaneous treatment of several diseases or move toward identification of a common target among the biological processes involved in aging. In this chapter, we will discuss some of the basic concepts of the role of ion channels in aging and will present an overview of the function of ion channels in some of the most common aging-related diseases.

Keywords: ion channels, aging, aging-related diseases, sinoatrial node, neurodegeneration, glaucoma, cancer

1. Introduction

Ion channels are pore membrane-associated proteins that allow movement of ionic fluxes between intracellular and extracellular fluids and within intracellular compartments. About

1.5% of the human genome encodes more than 400 ion channels. In addition, heteromerization and alternative splicing further increase functional diversity of ion channels [1–3].

Most ion channels are selective as they can discriminate between electrical charge and size of ions and they can allow unidirectional movement of only a specific ion (mostly K^+, Na^+, Ca^{2+}, or Cl^-) through the pore. Changes of ionic fluxes and, consequently, variations of electrical charge across membranes control virtually every cellular event including contraction, neuronal conductance, secretion, proliferation, and cell death. Therefore, abnormal changes of ionic gradients can underlie age-dependent decline of physiological functions. In addition, malfunction of ion channels is often associated with organ failure [4] during the process of aging.

In a resting state, ATP-driven pumps generate and maintain ionic gradients resulting in high intracellular K^+ (the most abundant intracellular ion) and low Na^+ and Ca^{2+}. In addition, the cytosolic surface membrane of all living cells is characterized by the accumulation of a net negative electrical charge than the extracellular surface of the membrane (membrane potential) that can range from −20 mV in epithelial nonexcitable cells to −100 mV in neurons. Because of this separation of electric charge and ionic concentrations across the membrane, opening of a Na^+ ion channel produces a flow of a positive charge (current, *i*) caused by the movement of Na^+ ions from the extracellular environment to the cytosol (Na^+ current, iNa^+). The augmented concentration of positive charges in the cytosol decreases the net negative charge with a process called depolarization. In plants, depolarization is achieved by an outward Cl^- flux.

In neurons and muscle cells, such as cardiac myocytes, depolarization is a critical event that underlies neuronal signaling and contraction. Depolarization activates more Na^+ (via a positive feedback), K^+, and Ca^{2+} channels and the respective ions will cross the membrane according to their electrochemical gradients. Therefore, K^+ leaving the cells will counteract depolarization, an event called repolarization. Inactivation of Na^+ and Ca^{2+} channels in combination with the outward fluxes of K^+ will produce the falling phase of the action potential which will continue until the ionic balances across the membranes are reestablished (resting phase). Each cell type presents a collection of ion channels that shape amplitude and duration of the action potential differently. For example, in neurons, changes of ionic fluxes occur very rapidly producing action potentials with fast depolarization and repolarization (lasting less than 1 ms) that propagates as unidirectional waves along the axon. Frequencies, duration, and amplitudes of action potentials produce neuronal signaling that guarantees transfer and elaboration of information from different body compartments, external to internal environment, and vice versa [5].

In the heart, action potentials are much slower (400 ms) than in neurons and they mostly serve the purpose to control contraction. This event is regulated by a collaborative effort between surface membrane and intracellular Ca^{2+} channels (ICCs) (e.g., ryanodine receptors, RyRs) in which the initial small amount of Ca^{2+} ions entering the cell from the extracellular environment bind and activate RyRs channels located on intracellular Ca^{2+} stores. This event, called Ca^{2+}-induced Ca^{2+} release, produces large changes of cytosolic Ca^{2+} concentration that is used by contracting fibers to produce motion and guarantee a conversion of an electrical stimulus into a mechanical response [6].

2. Ion channels in the aging mosaic of the sinoatrial node (SAN)

The sinoatrial node is a specialized bundle of neurons that innervate the heart and act as a "pacemaker" by generating electrical impulses at regular intervals that allow the heart to contract rhythmically. Typically, SAN dysfunction (SND) can be related to the use of specific medications (e.g., beta blockers) [7]; however, SAN function is known to decline during aging [8], resulting in pacemaker diseases in senior people. Unfortunately, SND can be corrected only by treating the extrinsic causes. Clinical manifestation of aging-dependent SND can be associated with a dramatic alteration of a series of parameters that can range from an increased action potential duration of the neurons composing the SAN to a reduction of the intrinsic heart rate [8] (IHR; defined as the rate at which the heart contracts without the contribution of the SAN and hormones). These phenomena are directly associated with changes in the activity of several ion channels that fail to control outward and inward ionic fluxes properly in the SAN and cardiac muscle. Interestingly, several study focusing on understanding age-dependent changes of gene expression revealed that expression of several channels are altered in the SAN and cardiac myocytes of aged animals. Perhaps counterintuitively, it was observed that in aged animals Na^+, Ca^{2+}, and K^+ channels increased their expression level in the SAN and atrial muscle [9–12].

It is predictable that an increased expression of Na^+ and Ca^{2+} channels would produce larger Na^+ and Ca^{2+} fluxes. The consequent increased cytosolic concentration of these two ions in neurons could explain the elongation of the aging-dependent action potential duration in the SAN because, for example, more time is required to remove Ca^{2+}. In contrast, increased K^+ currents would repolarize the cells faster and therefore increased K^+ efflux should accelerate the action potential duration.

Age-dependent changes of ion channel expression can also be specific to cardiac myocytes. For example, a significantly decreased RyR expression level has been found only in atrial cells that may be responsible for the age-dependent reduction of the IHR [9]. Furthermore, recent studies showed that an abnormal cytosolic Ca^{2+} concentration due to upregulation of the transient receptor potential vanilloid type 2 (TRPV2) calcium channel could cause alteration of posttranslational modification of progerin, which can contribute to the phenotype of premature aging linked to Hutchinson-Gilford progeria syndrome (HGPS) [13, 14].

3. Ion channels in the aging of the nervous system

The human nervous system is composed of two parts, the central nervous system (CNS) and the peripheral nervous system (PNS). Cells of the human nervous system mostly comprise neuronal cells, whose axons bundle in the PNS and nonneuronal cells such as glia cells, microglia, astrocytes, and oligodendrocytes. As any other cell, all cells of the nervous system are susceptible to aging and although aging dramatically increases the risk of developing cognitive disorders that are typical of the CNS such as Alzheimer's disease (AD) or PNS such as amyotrophic lateral sclerosis, only few elders contract these pathologies (www.alz.org;

www.pdf.org; www.alsa.org). This suggests that a purely genetic origin of these diseases linked to aging is unlikely as individuals can live for over 100 years without any overt behavioral sign of neurodegeneration. In addition, these diseases affect particular populations of cells in specific areas of the brain suggesting that perhaps aging is not the trigger of these diseases but only worsens preexisting conditions.

Changes in Ca^{2+} homeostasis have been linked to aging-dependent deterioration of neuronal activity [15–20]. However, it is not yet clear whether it is a decreased or increased cytosolic Ca^{2+} concentration that mediates its noxious effects on brain performance during aging. For example, Ca^{2+} channels have been found to be reduced in genetically modified mice with accelerated age-dependent decay in learning and memory [21, 22]. However, this conclusion is contradicted by another study in which it is demonstrated that a long-lasting intracellular Ca^{2+} might render neurons vulnerable to age [22]. Furthermore, elegant work by the Stutzmann laboratory reported an increase in type 2 RyR transcripts in brains with mild cognitive impairment compared to those with no cognitive impairment. In addition, they found a reduction in a specific type 2 RyR splice variant that is associated with antiapoptotic function in brains of patients with mild cognitive impairment and Alzheimer's disease [23].

3.1. Reactive oxygen species (ROS) and ion channels in aging

Although there is a considerably large amount of studies on aging-related neurodegenerative diseases, very little is known about the process of aging in normal neurons. Nevertheless, it is generally accepted that neurons of an aging brain are characterized by accumulation of reactive oxygen species over time that are probably generated by an altered target of rapamycin (TOR) pathway [24]. However, ROS has also a protective role in neurons but the mechanism that control the threshold to which ROS become toxic is still heavily debated.

The deleterious effects of free radicals on neuronal homeostasis can be attributed to the ability of these chemical species to interact with a large variety of targets such as DNA and lipids. However, recent research has brought to light that activity of several neuronal ion channels can significantly change upon chemical interaction with free radicals and that this event can be related to aberrant cognitive functions during aging. For example, oxidizing agents dramatically inhibit Na^+ channels activity without affecting the concentration of the channels at the surface membrane suggesting a direct effect of the agent on the Na^+ channel [25]. Inhibition of Na^+ channel activity dampens the ability to produce enough depolarization to generate an action potential and therefore affects the overall brain function.

Oxidation of K^+ channels that are expressed in brain neurons has been reported. For example, the activity of K^+ channels expressed in the hippocampus (which is the part of the brain that controls memory formation) can be increased by ROS [26] resulting in an inhibition of neuronal excitability and possibly incapacity to form or retain memory during aging. Interestingly, several studies have shown that ROS can increase or decrease cytosolic Ca^{2+} according to the type of Ca^{2+} channel analyzed. For example, oxidation of the "L-type" Ca^{2+} channel decreased Ca^{2+} currents [27]. However, the oxidative activity of β-amyloid protein ($A\beta$) produced in the brains of Alzheimer's patients increased the activity of L-type Ca^{2+} [28, 29], suggesting that distinct oxidative agents can exert different effects on Ca^{2+} homeostasis. In contrast, reducing agents have been reported to increase activity of the "T-type" calcium channel [30]. This suggests that ROS agents can increase cytosolic Ca^{2+} concentration and that this event can contribute to loss of neuronal function in aging. Inositol 1, 4, 5-trisphosphate (IP_3) receptors (IP_3Rs) and RyRs are the two major intracellular Ca^{2+} channels that release Ca^{2+} from neuronal intracellular stores such as the endoplasmic reticulum (ER).

Intracellular Ca^{2+} channels mediate numerous Ca^{2+}-dependent processes, including cellular growth and development, gene expression, and neurotransmission [31–40]. Therefore, it is not surprising that aberrant ICC function has been implicated in aging and several age-related pathologies including Alzheimer's disease, Huntington's disease (HD), and glaucoma [41–48]. Phosphatidylinositol and IP_3 levels are reduced in brains of patients with AD and the ensuing smaller number of IP_3 binding sites correlates with the number of amyloid plaques and neurofibrillary tangles [19–24]. Importantly, similar IP_3R dysfunction was found in in vitro models for AD including primary neuronal cultures from mouse models of AD [44, 49, 50] and cortical neurons exposed to β-amyloid protein [49]. These findings are particularly interesting, given the selective response of IP_3R to elevated levels of oxidative stress. IP_3R-mediated Ca^{2+} release was increased following activation of M3 muscarinic receptors under conditions of elevated oxidative stress [51]. Similarly, nonlethal oxidative stress in neuronal cells resulted in a selective upregulation at both the transcriptional and translational levels of type 2 IP_3Rs [52]. These channels exhibit the strongest affinity for the endogenous ligand, IP_3, and are preferentially expressed in the membranes of the nuclear envelope, where they mediate nuclear Ca^{2+} release [52–55]. This nuclear Ca^{2+} release is thought to control gene expression responsible for cellular survival and death pathways, and therefore, represents a promising drug target for neurodegenerative diseases [56]. This is exemplified by the recent finding that homocysteine-inducible, endoplasmic reticulum stress-inducible, ubiquitin-like domain member 1 (HERPUD1) is cytoprotective by preventing IP_3R-mediated Ca^{2+} transfer from the ER to mitochondria [57]. Analogously to IP_3Rs, several neurodegenerative and age-related disorders show RyR dysfunction contributing to disease pathology and progression. AD patients exhibit changes in neuronal RyR expression and in ryanodine binding that correlates with cognitive decline and $A\beta$ deposition [42].

3.2. Aging of the nonneuronal cells in the nervous system

The vast amount of cells in the brain is nonneuronal cells such as glia, microglia, astrocytes, and oligodendrocytes. These cells maintain homeostasis, form myelin, and, importantly, they can provide protection to the CNS and PNS as they act as the first and main form of neuronal immune defense. Microglia acts as the resident innate immune system in the brain as they respond to and propagate inflammatory signals (e.g., impending from PNS) by producing proinflammatory cytokines that ultimately can generate cognitive consequences. Several clinical and experimental studies reported that both increased oxidative stress and increased inflammation are (among others) hallmarks of brain aging [30, 58]. Remarkably, it has been found that activation of microglia is dependent on the expression of the Kv1.5 potassium channel and β-amyloid peptide induces expression of the Kv1.5 potassium channels in microglia [59–61]. This suggests that increased oxidative stress in aging could produce inflammation by upregulating K^+ channels in microglia and that alteration of ion channels could be one of the possible causes of aging-dependent decline of neuronal functions.

4. Ion channels and glaucoma

Glaucoma is an age-related, progressive optic neuropathy that manifests with pathological changes in the optic nerve, activation and remodeling of optic nerve head astrocytes (ONHAs), and slow progressive death of retinal ganglion cells, often leading to blindness. Although the exact pathophysiology is still not completely understood, there is evidence to support ischemic, mechanical, and inflammatory components. In an effort to protect the integrity of the optic nerve and prevent the loss of retinal ganglion cells, research efforts have recently concentrated on glioprotection approaches targeting ONHAs [62, 63]. Glia and neuronal cells alike utilize fine-tuned calcium signaling pathways to control physiological functions. Recent studies have revealed complex intracellular Ca^{2+} signaling pathways in primary ONHA culture [55] and for the first time described a differential distribution of type 2 IP_3Rs and type 2 RyRs in the ER and the membranes of the nuclear envelope. Hence, it is likely that these receptor subtypes activate specific Ca^{2+}-sensitive genes that determine cellular fate. Of particular interest for the role of aberrant Ca^{2+} signaling in glaucoma is the finding that exposure of ONHAs to elevated hydrostatic pressure, as a model for increased intraocular pressure in glaucoma, results in the differential upregulation of type 2 RyRs [64]. Given the nuclear membrane localization of type 2 RyRs in ONHAs [55], it is likely that RyR-mediated Ca^{2+} release differentially activates gene expression. Similar pathways of calcium signaling have been identified in astrocytes from other parts of the CNS and recently been reviewed in detail [65].

5. Ion channels and cancer

Cancer is a group of diseases that claim about 8.4 million lives every year (www.cancer.org). Although in the past decades, medical research has dramatically improved prevention, diagnosis, and treatment of cancer and despite being among the most preventable diseases, cancer remains a leading cause of death worldwide.

Virtually, cancer can develop in any tissue and although each cancer type can be characterized by its unique features, the basic mechanisms that generate cancers are similar in all forms of the diseases. In a normal and healthy tissue, cell proliferation and cell death are controlled by a very complex, timely, and integrated signaling network that includes a series of checkpoints to ensure proper division factors of the cell or death. Cancer originates from an uncontrolled proliferation of cells that evade cell death and can eventually invade and/or outspread into other body compartments (metastasis).

Cancer can be caused by a multitude of environmental factors that can be external such as smoking, sun exposure, and/or internal such as inherited faulty genes and/or infections.

http://dx.doi.org/10.5772/63951

Although there can be a significant difference in the prevalence of cancers among different societies, overall cancer can affect every human being. Accordingly, aging is the highest single risk factor for developing cancer [66]. Recently, several ion channels have been found to play a major role in maintaining homeostasis of nonexcitable cells (**Figure 1**).

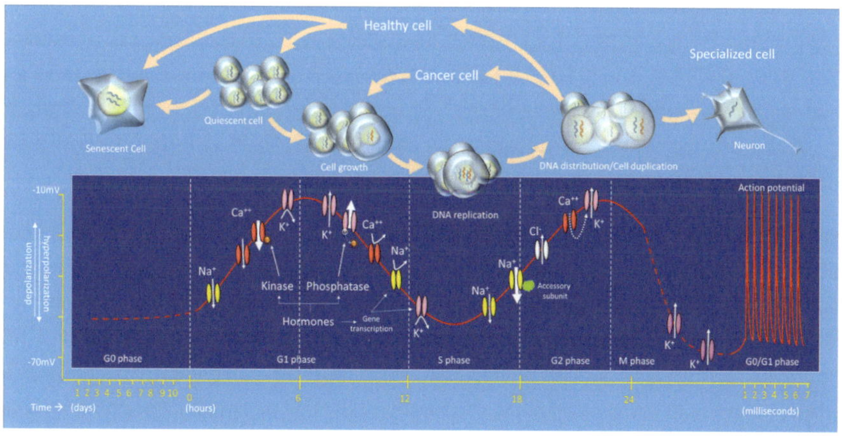

Figure 1. Schematic representation of the contribution of different ion channels to the membrane potential in function of time (e.g., nonexcitable cell vs. neuronal action potential). Overexpression and/or upregulation (e.g., via hormone-dependent regulation) of certain ion channels can contribute to suppress differentiation and increase duplication rate resulting in the generation of a cancerogenic phenotype.

In addition to the traditional role of allowing movements of ions across membranes, ion channels can also control mechanisms of transport, secretion, cell volume, and protein synthesis. For example, glucose transport is controlled by gradients of Na^+ [67, 68]. Furthermore, several transcription factors or proteins involved in secretory mechanism are activated by Ca^{2+} [69, 70]. Therefore, changes of intracellular ionic concentrations can regulate a variety of cellular event ranging from production of energy to protein synthesis, which are necessary for the ultimate process of cellular duplication. Several studies have reported that cancer cells of different histogenesis can express specific ion channels that can play an important role during proliferation [71].

One of the better characterized ion channels in cancer is the Kv11.1 (hERG1) potassium channel. This potassium channel is encoded by the human ether-a-go-go related gene 1 (hERG1), which has been found typically expressed in the mammalian heart in which it play a fundamental role in controlling repolarization and duration of action potential [72]. Remarkably, hERG1 channel has also been found expressed in different nonexcitable cancer cells but not in the organ from which the tumor has originated [73]. This suggests that the presence of this channel might provide a selective advantage to proliferation. Blockade or stimulation of hERG1 channel activity determined a strong inhibitory effect on cancer cell proliferation [74–78]. In addition, complete removal of the hERG1 protein from breast cancer cells determined death by activation of apoptosis [78]. These events indicate that the hERG1 is very important for cancer biology and its activity is kept under strict control.

Interestingly, the inhibitory effect on cell proliferation as a consequence of chronic stimulation of hERG1 channel was characterized by activation of a "cellular senescent program" [76, 79]. Senescent cells were initially described by Hayflick and Moorhead [80] as cells that have lost the ability to duplicate, though they may not die. Today, cellular senescence is defined as a permanent arrest of the cell cycle induced by a progressive increase of stresses [81–83]. At this time, it is not known what kind of stresses hERG1 agonists produce on cancer cells but their effect is mediated by permanent arrest of the cell cycle, increased expression of tumor suppressors (e.g., $p21^{waf/cif}$ and $p16^{INK4A}$) and decreased level of tumor markers (e.g., cyclins) resulting in a potent inhibition of cell proliferation [84–86]. This suggests that, by taking advantage of the ability to accelerate aging in cancer cells, hERG1 agonists could be used as an anticancer therapeutic strategy.

Other ion channels have been found playing fundamental roles in regulating biochemical signaling that underline important events in cancer biology which includes metastasis. Overtime, cancer cells acquire the ability to move and invade surrounding tissues by protruding membrane structures (invadopodia and pseudopodia) [87] through the intracellular space of the host organ. Remarkably, it has been discovered that ion channels are fundamental factors for regulation of invasion and migration of cancer cells. For example, the concerted activity of Ca^{2+}, K^+, and Cl channels that can exquisitely colocalize on the glioma surface membrane generates fluxes of ions and water that creates shrinkage of the membrane with consequent formation of invadopodia [88]. A direct consequence of this event is that cancer cells can move across tissue barriers (e.g., blood vessel) and colonize other body compartments. In addition, it has been shown that overexpression of Kv10 channels in which ion flux has been obstructed by a specific mutation did not lose the ability to promote cell proliferation [89, 90]. Although the mechanism through which this event occurs is not clearly understood, it appears that these channels can regulate activities of proteins that control proliferative cell signaling also when ion fluxes are not involved.

As hormones control most of the major organ functions by activating a variety of cellular signaling, it is not surprising that ion channels can be downstream effectors of hormone receptors. Growth of many cancers can depend on altered expression of hormone receptors. For example, high percentage of breast cancers are very sensitive to the action of insulin and/or sex hormones such as estrogen [91] or prostate cancer to testosterone [92]. Hormones can control ion channel activity by increasing their synthesis or by activating membrane signaling pathways (**Figure 1**). For example, hormones that bind G protein-coupled receptors (GPCR) produce release of the active $\beta\gamma$subunit of the heteromeric GTPase complex that ultimately binds and activates K^+ channels (e.g., GIRK). Alternatively, soluble hormone receptors can activate nongenomic signaling resulting in stimulation of kinases or phosphatases that modulate activity of ion channels by directly targeting these proteins [93–95]. Furthermore, as secretion is vastly controlled by intracellular changes in Ca^{2+} concentrations (e.g., Ca^{2+}-dependent insulin secretion), hormones must rely on ion channel function to be released in the body environment [96]. It is well established that with aging, organs become less sensitive to hormones. Although several examples of hormone-regulated ion channel activities have been proposed, knowledge on the role of these signalings in pathological conditions such as

http://dx.doi.org/10.5772/63951

cancer, age-related disease, and/or aging is very limited. Therefore, it appears that there is a compelling need to study the role of hormonal regulation of ion channels to better understand both aging and cancer.

6. Modulation of ion channels

Another level of complexity of regulation of ion channels is added by a number of modulatory proteins that have been shown to bind channels and alter their biophysical properties.

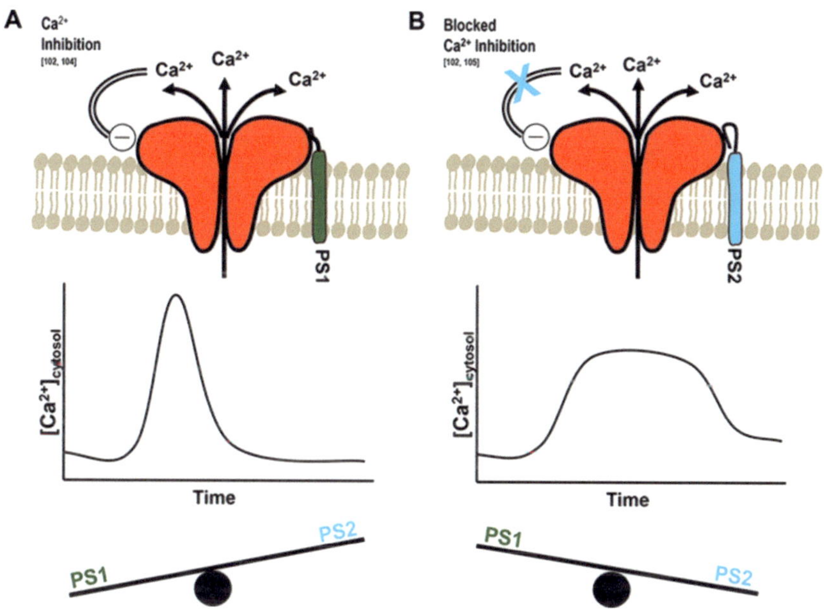

Figure 2. Presenilins differentially regulate RyR-mediated Ca^{2+} release.Representations of an individual RyR and its interaction with presenilin are shown in the top panels. Corresponding graphs below illustrate characteristics of Ca^{2+} transients mediated by RyR activity. Whole-cell cytosolic calcium concentrations (ordinate) are plotted over time (abscissa) to show the changes in the kinetics of Ca^{2+} transients dependent on presenilin binding to the RyR. Seesaws depict a predominant effect of presenilin 1 (PS1) over presenilin 2 PS2 or PS2 over PS1, as seen in young and aged animals, respectively [48]. (A) Binding of the PS1 N-terminal fragment to RyR increases open probability and results in heightened calcium release and fast channel inhibition by calcium at the RyR's inhibitory low affinity Ca^{2+} binding site. (B) Binding of PS2 to the RyR blocks inhibition at the low affinity Ca^{2+} binding site resulting in an increased duration of the Ca^{2+} transient.This figure was modified from reference [103], which was published under Open Access licence (©2015 by Andrew J. Payne *et al.*).

One of the best examples of involvement of ion channel modulation in aging includes Homer/Vesl proteins and the group of presenilins. The group of Homer proteins (reviewed in [97]) is a family of ubiquitously expressed scaffolding molecules. Through a conserved binding motif, Homer proteins interact with a number of synaptic proteins. Homer 1 proteins directly interact with IP_3Rs, RyRs, the group of transient receptor potential canonical (TRPC) channels, as well as mGluRs and some voltage-gated Ca^{2+} channels (reviewed in [97]). Intriguingly, in addition to enhancing synaptic transmission and providing a means of regulating excitability through tethering plasma membrane proteins to receptors and channels in the ER by formation of Homer tetramers, Homer proteins can alter the biophysical properties of their binding partners [98–100]. These interactions, especially with intracellular Ca^{2+} channels, have recently attracted increased interest due to their alterations in age-related diseases in the nervous system. For instance, in the aging brain, loss of the short isoform, Homer 1a, correlated with the loss of cognitive and motor function in mice [46]. Similarly, upregulation of the long isoform, Homer 1c, in the retina of glaucomatous mice showed a statistically significant association with severity of the disease phenotype and disease progression [47]. Furthermore, loss of Homer 1c immunoreactivity at glutamatergic synapses after experimental stroke was identified as a potential biomarker for early neurodegenerative processes, prior to initiation of apoptotic pathways [101]. Similarly, binding of presenilin proteins to RyRs results in a functional change of intracellular Ca^{2+} release [102–105]. Recent studies have demonstrated that altered levels of presenilin proteins in the aging brain correlate with the presence and severity of impairments in cognitive and motor function [48]; **Figure 2**), identifying the group of presenilins as putative drug target for neurodegeneration. In summary, intracellular Ca^{2+} channels are critical mediators of intracellular Ca^{2+} homeostasis and respond differentially to aging and pathological stimuli including oxidative stress. Furthermore, intracellular Ca^{2+} signaling is differentially regulated in various cell types and tissues and by a large number of modulators, providing a multitude of targets for pharmaceutical intervention in conditions characterized by neurodegeneration and aging.

7. Perspective

Aging is a process common to all living organisms that is associated with a progressive failure to adapt to changes in the environment. As ion channels are evolutionary conserved proteins that all cells of all living creatures utilize to sense and adapt to variations of both extracellular and intracellular environments, it is not surprising that malfunction of ion channels increases disease susceptibility that often simulates ailments of getting older. This suggests that drugs targeting ion channels can hold promise for treating aging. However, in consideration of the fact that more than 400 genes encoding for ion channels subunits have been identified so far, the role of ion channels in aging and aging-related diseases remains significantly underexplored. In addition, aging-dependent alteration of a particular ion channel appears to be organ and/or tissue-specific indicating that pharmacologic therapies targeting a specific ion channel should be tailored to a particular organ.

The ultimate consequence of all diseases is pain which appears to get worse with age and can have serious negative impact on quality of life. In recent time, a substantial increased awareness on the critical role of ion channels in diseases and pain has been achieved so that ion channels are emerging as novel therapeutic targets in the treatment of pain.

Acknowledgements

This material is the result of work supported with resources and the use of facilities at the Edward Hines Jr. VA Hospital, Hines, IL. The contents do not represent the views of the U.S. Department of Veterans Affairs or the United States Government. Additional support by the Dr. John P. and Therese E. Mulcahy Endowed Professorship in Ophthalmology (SK) and by the Cronk Family Foundation is gratefully acknowledged.

To Fiore e Rosa

Author details

Vidhya Rao[1], Simon Kaja[1,2,3] and Saverio Gentile[1*]

*Address all correspondence to: sagentile@lumc.edu

1 Department of Molecular Pharmacology and Therapeutics, Stritch School of Medicine, Loyola University Chicago, Maywood, Illinois, USA

2 Department of Ophthalmology, Stritch School of Medicine, Loyola University Chicago, Maywood, Illinois, USA

3 Research Service, Edward Hines Jr. Veterans Administration Hospital, Hines, Illinois, USA

References

[1] Lee A, Fakler B, Kaczmarek LK, Isom LL. (2014) More than a pore: ion channel signaling complexes. J Neurosci, 34, 15159–15169.

[2] Brueggemann LI, Gentile S, Byron KL. (2013) Social networking among voltage-activated potassium channels. Prog Mol Biol Transl Sci, 117, 269–302.

[3] Hille B. (1978) Ionic channels in excitable membranes. Current problems and biophysical approaches. Biophys J, 22, 283–294.

[4] Kass RS. (2005) The channelopathies: novel insights into molecular and genetic mechanisms of human disease. J Clin Invest, 115, 1986–1989.

[5] Bean BP. (2007) The action potential in mammalian central neurons. Nat Rev Neurosci, 8, 451–465.

[6] Amin AS, Tan HL, Wilde AA. (2010) Cardiac ion channels in health and disease. Heart Rhythm, 7, 117–126.

[7] Jensen PN, Gronroos NN, Chen LY, Folsom AR, deFilippi C, Heckbert SR, Alonso A. (2014) Incidence of and risk factors for sick sinus syndrome in the general population. J Am Coll Cardiol, 64, 531–538.

[8] Haqqani HM, Kalman JM. (2007) Aging and sinoatrial node dysfunction: musings on the not-so-funny side. Circulation, 115, 1178–1179.

[9] Tellez JO, McZewski M, Yanni J, Sutyagin P, Mackiewicz U, Atkinson A, Inada S, Beresewicz A, Billeter R, Dobrzynski H, Boyett MR. (2011) Ageing-dependent remodelling of ion channel and Ca2+ clock genes underlying sino-atrial node pacemaking. Exp Physiol, 96, 1163–1178.

[10] Tellez JO, Dobrzynski H, Greener ID, Graham GM, Laing E, Honjo H, Hubbard SJ, Boyett MR, Billeter R. (2006) Differential expression of ion channel transcripts in atrial muscle and sinoatrial node in rabbit. Circ Res, 99, 1384–1393.

[11] Larson ED, St Clair JR, Sumner WA, Bannister RA, Proenza C. (2013) Depressed pacemaker activity of sinoatrial node myocytes contributes to the age-dependent decline in maximum heart rate. Proc Natl Acad Sci U S A, 110, 18011–18016.

[12] Rose RA. (2011) Keeping the clocks ticking as we age: changes in sinoatrial node gene expression and function in the ageing heart. Exp Physiol, 96, 1114–1115.

[13] Kalinowski A, Qin Z, Coffey K, Kodali R, Buehler MJ, Losche M, Dahl KN. (2013) Calcium causes a conformational change in lamin A tail domain that promotes farnesyl-mediated membrane association. Biophys J, 104, 2246–2253.

[14] Lo CY, Tjong YW, Ho JC, Siu CW, Cheung SY, Tang NL, Yu S, Tse HF, Yao X. (2014) An upregulation in the expression of vanilloid transient potential channels 2 enhances hypotonicity-induced cytosolic Ca(2)(+) rise in human induced pluripotent stem cell model of Hutchinson-Gillford Progeria. PLoS One, 9, e87273.

[15] Feng Z, Zhang JT. (2000) Central nervous system calcium homeostasis imbalance and brain aging. Sheng Li Ke Xue Jin Zhan, 31, 102–108.

[16] Gibson GE, Peterson C. (1987) Calcium and the aging nervous system. Neurobiol Aging, 8, 329–343.

[17] Hartmann H, Eckert A, Muller WE. (1994) Disturbances of the neuronal calcium homeostasis in the aging nervous system. Life Sci, 55, 2011–2018.

[18] Khachaturian ZS. (1991) Calcium and the aging brain: upsetting a delicate balance? Geriatrics, 46, 78–79, 83.

[19] Khachaturian ZS. (1994) Calcium hypothesis of Alzheimer's disease and brain aging. Ann N Y Acad Sci, 747, 1–11.

[20] Thibault O, Gant JC, Landfield PW. (2007) Expansion of the calcium hypothesis of brain aging and Alzheimer's disease: minding the store. Aging Cell, 6, 307–317.

[21] Yamada S, Uchida S, Ohkura T, Kimura R, Yamaguchi M, Suzuki M, Yamamoto M. (1996) Alterations in calcium antagonist receptors and calcium content in senescent brain and attenuation by nimodipine and nicardipine. J Pharmacol Exp Ther, 277, 721–727.

[22] Giovannelli L, Pepeu G. (1989) Effect of age on K+–induced cytosolic Ca2+ changes in rat cortical synaptosomes. J Neurochem, 53, 392–398.

[23] Bruno AM, Huang JY, Bennett DA, Marr RA, Hastings ML, Stutzmann GE. (2012) Altered ryanodine receptor expression in mild cognitive impairment and Alzheimer's disease. Neurobiol Aging, 33, 1001 e1-6.

[24] Blagosklonny MV. (2008) Aging: ROS or TOR. Cell Cycle, 7, 3344–3354.

[25] Evans JR, Bielefeldt K. (2000) Regulation of sodium currents through oxidation and reduction of thiol residues. Neuroscience, 101, 229–236.

[26] Santarelli LC, Wassef R, Heinemann SH, Hoshi T. (2006) Three methionine residues located within the regulator of conductance for K+ (RCK) domains confer oxidative sensitivity to large-conductance Ca2+–activated K+ channels. J Physiol, 571, 329–348.

[27] Chiamvimonvat N, O'Rourke B, Kamp TJ, Kallen RG, Hofmann F, Flockerzi V, Marban E. (1995) Functional consequences of sulfhydryl modification in the pore-forming subunits of cardiovascular Ca2+ and Na+ channels. Circ Res, 76, 325–334.

[28] Foster TC, Sharrow KM, Masse JR, Norris CM, Kumar A. (2001) Calcineurin links Ca2+ dysregulation with brain aging. J Neurosci, 21, 4066–4073.

[29] Ueda K, Shinohara S, Yagami T, Asakura K, Kawasaki K. (1997) Amyloid beta protein potentiates Ca2+ influx through L-type voltage-sensitive Ca2+ channels: a possible involvement of free radicals. J Neurochem, 68, 265–271.

[30] Todorovic SM, Jevtovic-Todorovic V, Meyenburg A, Mennerick S, Perez-Reyes E, Romano C, Olney JW, Zorumski CF. (2001) Redox modulation of T-type calcium channels in rat peripheral nociceptors. Neuron, 31, 75–85.

[31] Bading H. (2000) Transcription-dependent neuronal plasticity the nuclear calcium hypothesis. Eur J Biochem, 267, 5280–5283.

[32] Hardingham GE, Chawla S, Johnson CM, Bading H. (1997) Distinct functions of nuclear and cytoplasmic calcium in the control of gene expression. Nature, 385, 260–265.

[33] Kelly PT, Mackinnon RL, 2nd, Dietz RV, Maher BJ, Wang J. (2005) Postsynaptic IP3 receptor-mediated Ca2+ release modulates synaptic transmission in hippocampal neurons. Brain Res Mol Brain Res, 135, 232–248.

[34] Liu Q, Chen B, Yankova M, Morest DK, Maryon E, Hand AR, Nonet ML, Wang ZW. (2005) Presynaptic ryanodine receptors are required for normal quantal size at the Caenorhabditis elegans neuromuscular junction. J Neurosci, 25, 6745–6754.

[35] Simkus CR, Stricker C. (2002) The contribution of intracellular calcium stores to mEPSCs recorded in layer II neurones of rat barrel cortex. J Physiol, 545, 521–535.

[36] Suryanarayanan A, Slaughter MM. (2006) Synaptic transmission mediated by internal calcium stores in rod photoreceptors. J Neurosci, 26, 1759–1766.

[37] Unni VK, Zakharenko SS, Zablow L, DeCostanzo AJ, Siegelbaum SA. (2004) Calcium release from presynaptic ryanodine-sensitive stores is required for long-term depression at hippocampal CA3-CA3 pyramidal neuron synapses. J Neurosci, 24, 9612–9622.

[38] West AE, Chen WG, Dalva MB, Dolmetsch RE, Kornhauser JM, Shaywitz AJ, Takasu MA, Tao X, Greenberg ME. (2001) Calcium regulation of neuronal gene expression. Proc Natl Acad Sci U S A, 98, 11024–11031.

[39] Mathew SS, Hablitz JJ. (2008) Calcium release via activation of presynaptic IP3 receptors contributes to kainate-induced IPSC facilitation in rat neocortex. Neuropharmacology, 55, 106–116.

[40] Dropic AJ, Brailoiu E, Cooper RL. (2005) Presynaptic mechanism of action induced by 5-HT in nerve terminals: possible involvement of ryanodine and IP3 sensitive 2+ stores. Comp Biochem Physiol A Mol Integr Physiol, 142, 355–361.

[41] Bezprozvanny I, Hayden MR. (2004) Deranged neuronal calcium signaling and Huntington disease. Biochem Biophys Res Commun, 322, 1310–1317.

[42] Kelliher M, Fastbom J, Cowburn RF, Bonkale W, Ohm TG, Ravid R, Sorrentino V, O'Neill C. (1999) Alterations in the ryanodine receptor calcium release channel correlate with Alzheimer's disease neurofibrillary and beta-amyloid pathologies. Neuroscience, 92, 499–513.

[43] Smith IF, Hitt B, Green KN, Oddo S, LaFerla FM. (2005) Enhanced caffeine-induced Ca2+ release in the 3xTg-AD mouse model of Alzheimer's disease. J Neurochem, 94, 1711–1718.

[44] Stutzmann GE, Caccamo A, LaFerla FM, Parker I. (2004) Dysregulated IP3 signaling in cortical neurons of knock-in mice expressing an Alzheimer's-linked mutation in presenilin1 results in exaggerated Ca2+ signals and altered membrane excitability. J Neurosci, 24, 508–513.

[45] Ziegler SI, Haberkorn U, Byrne H, Tong C, Kaja S, Richolt JA, Byrne H, Tong C, Schosser R, Krieter H, Kaja S, Richolt JA, Lammertsma AA, Price P. (1996) Measurement of liver blood flow using oxygen-15 labelled water and dynamic positron emission tomography: limitations of model description. Eur J Nucl Med, 23, 169–177.

[46] Kaja S, Sumien N, Borden PK, Khullar N, Iqbal M, Collins JL, Forster MJ, Koulen P. (2013) Homer-1a immediate early gene expression correlates with better cognitive performance in aging. Age (Dordr), 35, 1799–1808.

http://dx.doi.org/10.5772/63951

[47] Kaja S, Naumchuk Y, Grillo SL, Borden PK, Koulen P. (2014) Differential up-regulation of Vesl-1/Homer 1 protein isoforms associated with decline in visual performance in a preclinical glaucoma model. Vision Res, 94, 16–23.

[48] Kaja S, Sumien N, Shah VV, Puthawala I, Maynard AN, Khullar N, Payne AJ, Forster MJ, Koulen P. (2015) Loss of spatial memory, learning, and motor function during normal aging is accompanied by changes in brain presenilin 1 and 2 expression levels. Mol Neurobiol, 52, 545–554.

[49] Ferreiro E, Resende R, Costa R, Oliveira CR, Pereira CM. (2006) An endoplasmic-reticulum-specific apoptotic pathway is involved in prion and amyloid-beta peptides neurotoxicity. Neurobiol Dis, 23, 669–678.

[50] Kasri NN, Kocks SL, Verbert L, Hebert SS, Callewaert G, Parys JB, Missiaen L, De Smedt H. (2006) Up-regulation of inositol 1,4,5-trisphosphate receptor type 1 is responsible for a decreased endoplasmic-reticulum Ca2+ content in presenilin double knock-out cells. Cell Calcium, 40, 41–51.

[51] Tang TH, Chang CT, Wang HJ, Erickson JD, Reichard RA, Martin AG, Shannon EK, Martin AL, Huang YW, Aronstam RS. (2013) Oxidative stress disruption of receptor-mediated calcium signaling mechanisms. J Biomed Sci, 20, 48.

[52] Kaja S, Duncan RS, Longoria S, Hilgenberg JD, Payne AJ, Desai NM, Parikh RA, Burroughs SL, Gregg EV, Goad DL, Koulen P. (2011) Novel mechanism of increased Ca2+ release following oxidative stress in neuronal cells involves type 2 inositol-1,4,5-trisphosphate receptors. Neuroscience, 175, 281–291.

[53] Leite MF, Thrower EC, Echevarria W, Koulen P, Hirata K, Bennett AM, Ehrlich BE, Nathanson MH. (2003) Nuclear and cytosolic calcium are regulated independently. Proc Natl Acad Sci U S A, 100, 2975–2980.

[54] Duncan RS, Hwang SY, Koulen P. (2007) Differential inositol 1,4,5-trisphosphate receptor signaling in a neuronal cell line. Int J Biochem Cell Biol, 39, 1852–1862.

[55] Kaja S, Payne AJ, Patel KR, Naumchuk Y, Koulen P. (2015) Differential subcellular Ca2+ signaling in a highly specialized subpopulation of astrocytes. Exp Neurol, 265, 59–68.

[56] Duncan RS, Goad DL, Grillo MA, Kaja S, Payne AJ, Koulen P. (2010) Control of intracellular calcium signaling as a neuroprotective strategy. Molecules, 15, 1168–1195.

[57] Paredes F, Parra V, Torrealba N, Navarro-Marquez M, Gatica D, Bravo-Sagua R, Troncoso R, Pennanen C, Quiroga C, Chiong M, Caesar C, Taylor WR, Molgo J, San Martin A, Jaimovich E, Lavandero S. (2016) HERPUD1 protects against oxidative stress-induced apoptosis through downregulation of the inositol 1,4,5-trisphosphate receptor. Free Radic Biol Med, 90, 206–218.

[58] Joseph JA, Shukitt-Hale B, Casadesus G, Fisher D. (2005) Oxidative stress and inflammation in brain aging: nutritional considerations. Neurochem Res, 30, 927–935

[59] Jou I, Pyo H, Chung S, Jung SY, Gwag BJ, Joe EH. (1998) Expression of Kv1.5 K+ channels in activated microglia in vivo. Glia, 24, 408–414.

[60] Pannasch U, Farber K, Nolte C, Blonski M, Yan Chiu S, Messing A, Kettenmann H. (2006) The potassium channels Kv1.5 and Kv1.3 modulate distinct functions of microglia. Mol Cell Neurosci, 33, 401–411.

[61] Chung S, Lee J, Joe EH, Uhm DY. (2001) Beta-amyloid peptide induces the expression of voltage dependent outward rectifying K+ channels in rat microglia. Neurosci Lett, 300, 67–70.

[62] Kaja S, Payne AJ, Naumchuk Y, Levy D, Zaidi DH, Altman AM, Nawazish S, Ghuman JK, Gerdes BC, Moore MA, Koulen P. (2015) Plate reader-based cell viability assays for glioprotection using primary rat optic nerve head astrocytes. Exp Eye Res, 138, 159–166.

[63] Kaja S, Payne AJ, Singh T, Ghuman JK, Sieck EG, Koulen P. (2015) An optimized lactate dehydrogenase release assay for screening of drug candidates in neuroscience. J Pharmacol Toxicol Methods, 73, 1–6.

[64] Mandal A, Shahidullah M, Delamere NA. (2010) Hydrostatic pressure-induced release of stored calcium in cultured rat optic nerve head astrocytes. Invest Ophthalmol Vis Sci, 51, 3129–3138.

[65] Bazargani N, Attwell D. (2016) Astrocyte calcium signaling: the third wave. Nat Neurosci, 19, 182–189.

[66] Finkel T, Serrano M, Blasco MA. (2007) The common biology of cancer and ageing. Nature, 448, 767–774.

[67] Wright EM. (2001) Renal Na(+)-glucose cotransporters. Am J Physiol Renal Physiol, 280, F10-8.

[68] Wright EM, Hirayama BA, Loo DF. (2007) Active sugar transport in health and disease. J Intern Med, 261, 32–43.

[69] Hogan PG, Chen L, Nardone J, Rao A. (2003) Transcriptional regulation by calcium, calcineurin, and NFAT. Genes Dev, 17, 2205–2232.

[70] Johnson CM, Hill CS, Chawla S, Treisman R, Bading H. (1997) Calcium controls gene expression via three distinct pathways that can function independently of the Ras/mitogen-activated protein kinases (ERKs) signaling cascade. J Neurosci, 17, 6189–6202.

[71] Rao VR, Perez-Neut M, Kaja S, Gentile S. Voltage-gated ion channels in cancer cell proliferation. Cancers (Basel), 7, 849–875.

[72] Vandenberg JI, Perry MD, Perrin MJ, Mann SA, Ke Y, Hill AP. (2012) hERG K(+) channels: structure, function, and clinical significance. Physiol Rev, 92, 1393–1478.

[73] Arcangeli A. (2005) Expression and role of hERG channels in cancer cells. Novartis Found Symp, 266, 225–232; discussion 232–234.

[74] Ganapathi SB, Kester M, Elmslie KS. (2009) State-dependent block of HERG potassium channels by R-roscovitine: implications for cancer therapy. Am J Physiol Cell Physiol, 296, C701-10.

[75] Glassmeier G, Hempel K, Wulfsen I, Bauer CK, Schumacher U, Schwarz JR. (2012) Inhibition of HERG1 K+ channel protein expression decreases cell proliferation of human small cell lung cancer cells. Pflugers Arch, 463, 365–376.

[76] Lansu K, Gentile S. Potassium channel activation inhibits proliferation of breast cancer cells by activating a senescence program. Cell Death Dis, 4, e652.

[77] Perez-Neut M, Rao VR, Gentile S. hERG1/Kv11.1 activation stimulates transcription of p21waf/cip in breast cancer cells via a calcineurin-dependent mechanism. Oncotarget.

[78] Perez-Neut M, Shum A, Cuevas BD, Miller R, Gentile S. Stimulation of hERG1 channel activity promotes a calcium-dependent degradation of cyclin E2, but not cyclin E1, in breast cancer cells. Oncotarget, 6, 1631–1639.

[79] Hayflick L, Moorhead PS. (1961) The serial cultivation of human diploid cell strains. Exp Cell Res, 25, 585–621.

[80] Campisi J. (2000) Cancer, aging and cellular senescence. In Vivo, 14, 183–188.

[81] Munoz-Espin D, Serrano M. (2014) Cellular senescence: from physiology to pathology. Nat Rev Mol Cell Biol, 15, 482–496.

[82] Rodier F, Campisi J. (2011) Four faces of cellular senescence. J Cell Biol, 192, 547–556.

[83] Lansu K, Gentile S. (2013) Potassium channel activation inhibits proliferation of breast cancer cells by activating a senescence program. Cell Death Dis, 4, e652.

[84] Perez-Neut M, Rao VR, Gentile S. (2014) hERG1/Kv11.1 activation stimulates transcription of p21waf/cip in breast cancer cells via a calcineurin-dependent mechanism. Oncotarget.

[85] Perez-Neut M, Shum A, Cuevas BD, Miller R, Gentile S. (2014) Stimulation of hERG1 channel activity promotes a calcium-dependent degradation of cyclin E2, but not cyclin E1, in breast cancer cells. Oncotarget, 6, 1631–1639.

[86] Leong HS, Robertson AE, Stoletov K, Leith SJ, Chin CA, Chien AE, Hague MN, Ablack A, Carmine-Simmen K, McPherson VA, Postenka CO, Turley EA, Courtneidge SA, Chambers AF, Lewis JD. (2014) Invadopodia are required for cancer cell extravasation and are a therapeutic target for metastasis. Cell Rep, 8, 1558–1570.

[87] Sontheimer H. (2008) An unexpected role for ion channels in brain tumor metastasis. Exp Biol Med (Maywood), 233, 779–791.

[88] Pardo LA, del Camino D, Sanchez A, Alves F, Bruggemann A, Beckh S, Stuhmer W. (1999) Oncogenic potential of EAG K(+) channels. EMBO J, 18, 5540–5547.

[89] Wu X, Zhong D, Lin B, Zhai W, Ding Z, Wu J. (2013) p38 MAPK regulates the expression of ether a go-go potassium channel in human osteosarcoma cells. Radiol Oncol, 47, 42–49.

[90] Hassan MS, Ansari J, Spooner D, Hussain SA. (2010) Chemotherapy for breast cancer (Review). Oncol Rep, 24, 1121–1131.

[91] Michaud JE, Billups KL, Partin AW. (2015) Testosterone and prostate cancer: an evidence-based review of pathogenesis and oncologic risk. Ther Adv Urol, 7, 378–387.

[92] Gentile S, Darden T, Erxleben C, Romeo C, Russo A, Martin N, Rossie S, Armstrong DL. (2006) Rac GTPase signaling through the PP5 protein phosphatase. Proc Natl Acad Sci U S A, 103, 5202–5206.

[93] Simoncini T, Genazzani AR. (2003) Non-genomic actions of sex steroid hormones. Eur J Endocrinol, 148, 281–292.

[94] Storey NM, Gentile S, Ullah H, Russo A, Muessel M, Erxleben C, Armstrong DL. (2006) Rapid signaling at the plasma membrane by a nuclear receptor for thyroid hormone. Proc Natl Acad Sci U S A, 103, 5197–5201.

[95] Draznin B. (1988) Intracellular calcium, insulin secretion, and action. Am J Med, 85, 44–58.

[96] Kaja S, Payne AJ, Burroughs SL, Koulen P. (2013) Homer. In: Encyclopedia of Signaling Molecules (ed. S Choi). Springer.

[97] Westhoff JH, Hwang SY, Duncan RS, Ozawa F, Volpe P, Inokuchi K, Koulen P. (2003) Vesl/Homer proteins regulate ryanodine receptor type 2 function and intracellular calcium signaling. Cell Calcium, 34, 261–269.

[98] Duncan RS, Hwang SY, Koulen P. (2005) Effects of Vesl/Homer proteins on intracellular signaling. Exp Biol Med (Maywood), 230, 527–535.

[99] Hwang SY, Wei J, Westhoff JH, Duncan RS, Ozawa F, Volpe P, Inokuchi K, Koulen P. (2003) Differential functional interaction of two Vesl/Homer protein isoforms with ryanodine receptor type 1: a novel mechanism for control of intracellular calcium signaling. Cell Calcium, 34, 177–184.

[100] Kaja S, Yang SH, Wei J, Fujitani K, Liu R, Brun-Zinkernagel AM, Simpkins JW, Inokuchi K, Koulen P. (2003) Estrogen protects the inner retina from apoptosis and ischemia-induced loss of Vesl-1L/Homer 1c immunoreactive synaptic connections. Invest Ophthalmol Vis Sci, 44, 3155–3162.

[101] Payne AJ, Gerdes BC, Naumchuk Y, McCalley AE, Kaja S, Koulen P. (2013) Presenilins regulate the cellular activity of ryanodine receptors differentially through isotype-specific N-terminal cysteines. Exp Neurol, 250, 143–150.

[102] Payne AJ, Kaja S, Koulen P. (2015) Regulation of ryanodine receptor-mediated calcium signaling by presenilins. Receptors Clin Investig, 2, e449.

[103] Rybalchenko V, Hwang SY, Rybalchenko N, Koulen P. (2008) The cytosolic N-terminus of presenilin-1 potentiates mouse ryanodine receptor single channel activity. Int J Biochem Cell Biol, 40, 84–97.

[104] Hayrapetyan V, Rybalchenko V, Rybalchenko N, Koulen P. (2008) The N-terminus of presenilin-2 increases single channel activity of brain ryanodine receptors through direct protein-protein interaction. Cell Calcium, 44, 507–518.27.

[105] Chiamvimonvat N, O'Rourke B, Kamp TJ, Kallen RG, Hofmann F, Flockerzi V, Marban E. (1995) Functional consequences of sulfhydryl modification in the pore-forming subunits of cardiovascular Ca2+ and Na+ channels. Circ Res, 76, 325–334.

Chapter 4

Molecular Mechanisms of Skin Aging and Rejuvenation

Miri Kim and Hyun Jeong Park

Additional information is available at the end of the chapter

http://dx.doi.org/10.5772/62983

Abstract

The aging process in the skin is complex and influenced by more intrinsic and extrinsic factors than any other body organ. The effects of these two types of factors overlap for the most part. The combined effects of these two aging processes also affect dermal matrix alterations. The main clinical signs of skin aging include wrinkling and irregular pigmentation, which are influenced by a combination of intrinsic and extrinsic (e.g., UV radiation, heat, smoking, and pollutants) factors. Histologically, collagen decreases, and the dermis is replaced by abnormal elastic fibers as a cause of wrinkle formation through the loss of skin elasticity. There have been numerous studies of skin aging performed to elucidate the underlying molecular mechanisms and to develop various antiaging therapeutics and preventive strategies. We summarized the molecular mechanisms and treatments of skin aging. Mainly UV radiation induces ROS formation and DNA damage, leading to increased production of MMPs and decreased production of collagen in keratinocytes and fibroblasts, which reflect the central aspects of skin aging. Besides UV radiation exposure, extrinsic factors including tobacco smoking, exposure to environmental pollutants, infrared radiation, and heat contribute to premature skin aging. Like UV radiation, these factors cause ROS formation and increase expression of MMPs, thus accelerating skin aging by inducing extracellular matrix (ECM) degradation. Accumulated collagen fibrils inhibit the new collagen synthesis and account for the further degradation of the ECM through this positive feedback loop. Accumulating evidence for molecular mechanisms of skin aging should provide clinicians with an expanding spectrum of therapeutic targets in the treatment of skin aging.

Keywords: skin aging, photoaging, molecular mechanisms, antiaging treatments, rejuvenation

1. Introduction

Skin aging is a complex process affected by both genetic and environmental factors, and it is largely influenced by the cumulative damage from exposure to ultraviolet (UV) radiation. Chronic exposure of UV radiation on human skin leads to solar elastosis, degradation of the extracellular matrix (ECM), and wrinkle formation. Skin aging is affected by both intrinsic and extrinsic factors. Intrinsic or chronological skin aging results from the passage of time and is influenced by genetic factors. Extrinsic skin aging mainly results from UV irradiation, which is called photoaging. These two types of aging processes are superimposed in sun-exposed skin, and they have common clinical features caused by dermal matrix alterations that mainly contribute to wrinkle formation, laxity, and fragility of aged skin [1]. The dermal matrix contains ECM proteins such as collagen, elastin, and proteoglycans which is responsible for conferring strength and resiliency of the skin. Skin aging associated with dermal matrix alterations and atrophy can be caused by senescence of dermal cells such as fibroblasts, and decreased synthesis and accelerated breakdown of dermal collagen fibers [2]. Mouse models of skin aging have been developed extensively to elucidate intrinsic aging and photoaging processes, to validate *in vitro* biochemical data, and to test the effects of pharmacological tools for retarding skin aging because they have the advantages of being genetically similar to humans and are easily available. This review is focused on the molecular mechanisms of skin aging and antiaging treatment with a brief summary of the clinical and histological features of skin aging (**Figure 1**).

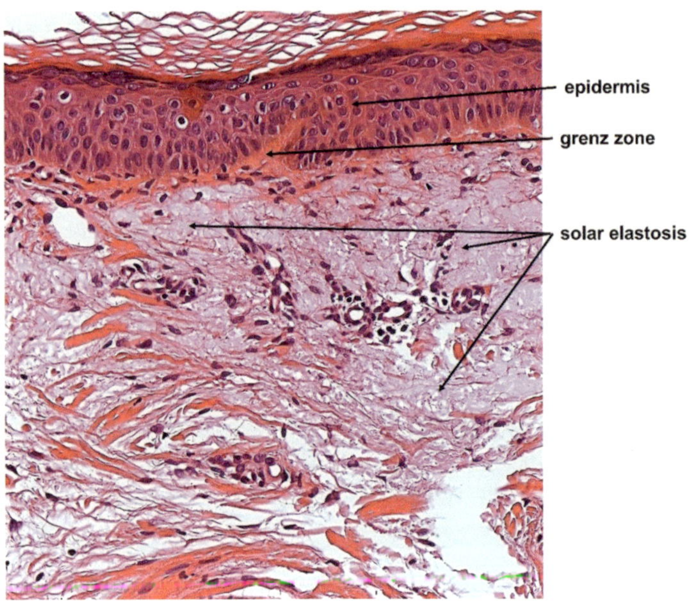

Figure 1. Histology of photoaged skin. The predominant histological finding of photodamaged skin is solar elastosis, which is basophilic degeneration of elastotic fibers in the dermis. Solar elastosis separates from the epidermis by a narrow band of normal-appearing collagen (grenz zone) with collagen fibers arranged horizontally (H&E stating. Original magnification ×400).

2. Clinical manifestations of chronological aging and photoaging

Clinical features of skin aging vary among individuals with differences in both genetic factors and lifestyles, which result in various degrees of cutaneous outcomes. Clinical signs of chronological aging include thinning of the skin, cigarette paper-like wrinkles, xerosis, loss of elasticity, and development of benign vascular formations such as cherry angiomas and benign overgrowths such as seborrheic keratosis [3]. Chronological aging is mainly the result of loss of soft tissue volume from fat atrophy, gravity-induced soft tissue redistribution, and weakened facial skeletal support related to bone resorption [3]. Clinical signs of photoaging include wrinkling, laxity, and a leather-like appearance, which are mainly the result of structural changes in the connective tissue of the dermis. These changes include both enzymatic degradation and reduced de novo synthesis of collagen, which cause wrinkling of the skin. The cumulative UV irradiation dose and Fitzpatrick skin type are used to assign the degree of photoaging. Individuals with Fitzpatrick skin types I and II show atrophic skin changes with fewer wrinkles, focal depigmentation, dysplastic premalignant changes such as actinic keratosis and malignant skin cancer. By contrast, skin types III and IV skin display hypertrophic features with deep wrinkles, leathery appearance, and lentigines [4]. In addition, photoaging includes changes in the dermal vascular structure, which appear clinically as telangiectasia (**Figure 2**).

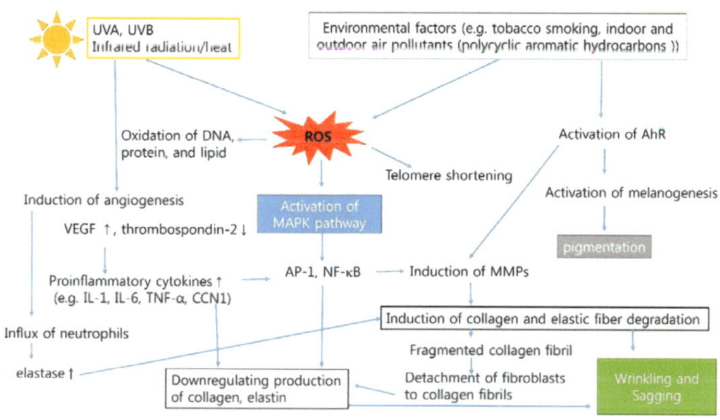

Figure 2. Schematic representation of pathogenesis of premature/extrinsic skin aging. ROS: reactive oxygen species, AhR: arylhydrocarbon receptor, NF-kB: nuclear factor kappa-B, IL-1: interleukin-1, TNF-α: tumor necrosis factor, CCN1: cysteine-rich protein 61, MAPK: mitogen-activated protein kinase, AP-1: activator protein 1, and MMPs: matrix metalloproteinases.

3. Histology of chronological aging and photoaging

Histological changes in chronologically aged skin are characterized by epidermal atrophy with reduced amounts of fibroblasts and collagen content in the dermis. The epidermal atrophy of intrinsically aged skin, which particularly affects the stratum spinosum, is related to lower epidermal turnover rate because of prolonged cell cycles [5]. Several studies of skin aging have reported that the epidermis is hypocellular with decreased melanocytes, mast cells, and Langerhans cells [6]. After the age of 30 years, the number of melanocytes decreases by 8–20% per decade [7]. The number of Langerhans cells in the epidermis becomes markedly decreased with noticeable morphological alterations and functional impairment. In dermis of chronologically aged skin, the collagen fibers are loose, thin, and disorganized compared with those in the sun-protected skin of young people [8]. The dermis of chronologically aged skin shows fewer mast cells and fibroblasts than that of young skin, and the amounts of collagen and elastic fibers are decreased [9]. In a study of the chronological changes in collagen fibers, the synthesis of collagen was found to be decreased by 30% in the first 4 years of menopause, then by 2% per year [10].

Photoaging causes several histological changes in the skin that are distinct from histological alterations that occur intrinsically during aging. In photoaging, the thickness of the epidermis and the morphology of epidermal is heterogeneous [11]. The epidermis of photodamaged skin is thicker than that of intrinsically aged skin, whereas the epidermis of severely photodamaged skin elicits epidermal atrophy [12]. Furthermore, increased numbers of atypical melanocytes and keratinocytes may be seen [4]. Melanogenesis is also upregulated and participates in the neutralization of free radicals induced by UV radiation exposure, which may act as a mechanism for protection from photodamage [13]. Major alterations of photoaged skin and their molecular effects occur primarily within the dermis and the dermoepidermal junction. There is an increased amount of glycosaminoglycans and proteoglycans within the aged dermis, possibly because of a rise in the level of matrix metalloproteinases (MMPs) with increased numbers of hyperplastic fibroblasts [14]. Unlike the hypocellular feature of chronologically aged skin, photoaged skin can present an increased number of inflammatory cells such as mast cells, eosinophils, and mononuclear cells [15]. In addition, the amount of extracellular matrix is decreased and breakdown of collagen fibers is increased, which may appear as wrinkles [16]. Meanwhile, the most pronounced histological feature of photoaging is the disintegration of elastic fibers (solar elastosis), which results in accumulation of amorphous, thickened, curled, and fragmented elastic fibers [17]. Elastotic material consists of elastin, fibrillin, glycosaminoglycans, particularly hyaluronic acid and versican, a large chondroitin sulfate proteoglycan. The pathogenesis of solar elastosis is assumed to be a result of both degradation and de novo synthesis, although it is not yet fully understood [18].

4. Molecular mechanisms of skin aging

4.1. Telomere shortening

Telomeres are tandem repeats of TTAGGG located at the distal ends of most eukaryotic organisms to protect chromosomes from degradation and from fusion with neighboring chromosomes [19]. Telomere shortening prevents aberrant cellular proliferation by limiting cellular division. A consequence of this protection is cellular senescence and aging [20]. Telomerase, also called telomere terminal transferase, is capable of adding the telomeric sequence TTAGGG to the 3′ end of telomeres [21]. In humans, telomerase plays a significant role in the maintenance of skin aging and oncogenesis [22]. The regulation of telomerase activity may therefore have significant role in antiaging and anticancer therapy. Gradual shortening of telomeres can explain cellular senescence that is essentially caused by intrinsic aging because it results from cell division. However, UV radiation exposure may induce telomere shortening by producing reactive oxygen species (ROS) in the skin [23]. Because UV radiation induces the formation of ROS in the skin and telomere shortening is accelerated by ROS, it has been postulated that skin exposed to UV radiation may have shorter telomeres compared with skin protected from UV radiation [1, 23]. Oikawa et al. [23] demonstrated that UVA irradiation accelerated telomere shortening in human cultured fibroblast cell lines by site-specific DNA damage at the GGG sequence in the telomere sequence. By contrast, Sugimoto et al. reported that telomere length in the epidermis and dermis was reduced with age and telomere length was not significantly different between epidermis from sun-exposed and sun-protected areas. They could not confirm that telomere shortening was associated with photoaging [19]. Telomeres are metabolically active and possess a set of characteristics *in vitro* and *in vivo*, which are known as biomarkers of aging and cellular senescence. Among biomarkers of cellular senescence, telomere shortening is a rather elegant and frequently used biomarker. The validity of telomere shortening as a marker for cellular senescence is based on the theoretical and experimental data. Further studies to determine the relationships between telomere restriction fragment length in skin cells and lifestyle/genetic background are necessary to confirm the validity of this marker. The details of molecular events and especially the function of telomere shortening in skin aging are not understood completely. However, interesting and important research progress is expected because advances in this field of research are mostly recent (**Table 1**).

Clinical	Histological	Molecular mechanism
Roughness	Increased compaction of stratum corneum, increased thickness of granular cell layer, reduced epidermal thickness and reduced epidermal mucin content	Decreased hyaluronan which plays an essential role in supporting tissue architecture and is also known as important factors to protect skin from dryness by its capacity to bind water
Irregular pigmentation		
Freckle	Reduced or increased number of hypertrophic, strongly dopa-positive melanocytes	
Solar lentigines	Elongation of epidermal rete ridges; increases in number and melanization of melanocytes	Mutations of keratinocyte and melanocyte genes which play a role in pigment formation and transfer. Stem cell factor mutations in keratinocyte have been suggested

Clinical	Histological	Molecular mechanism
		to be responsible for the development of solar lentigine
Guttate hypomelanosis	Decreased dopa oxidase-positive, KIT+, and melanocyte sand reduction in melanocytes	
Wrinkles	Thinned epidermis as well as less elastotic changes, tropoelastin, and collagen VII when compared to the surrounding photoaged skin	UVB radiation, infrared radiation, and heat produce and increase inflammatory cytokines, such as IL-1α, IL-6, and TNFα, which stimulate keratinocytes and dermal fibroblasts to produce matrix metalloproteinases (MMPs), leading to the degradation of extracellular matrix proteins and induction of wrinkles destruction of collagen and elastic fibers, and formation of wrinkles in sun-exposed skin. The expression of MMP-1 and MMP3 mRNA and protein levels is increased in dermal fibroblasts by the activation of ERK and JNK
Sagging	Loss of elastic tissue in the dermis and the remaining fibers were disorganized, shortened, and fragmented	UV radiation exposure causes keratinocytes to secrete GM-CSF, which triggers fibroblasts and stimulate the gene expression of MMP-1 to a greater extent than neprilysin by dermal fibroblasts and the secretion of IL-6, leading predominantly to sagging of the skin via the degradation of collagen I fibers by the enhanced activity of MMP-1
Inelasticity	Accumulated large amounts of homogenization and a dark blue amorphous elastotic material in the dermis, so-called solar elastosis	UV radiation, infrared radiation, and heat lead to an influx of neutrophils, which are packed with proteolytic enzymes (such as neutrophil elastase) that participate in extracellular matrix damage processes,

Clinical	Histological	Molecular mechanism
		mainly collagen and elastic fibers degradation. Neutrophil elastase is strongly associated with the development of solar elastosis resulting from continued exposure to UV radiation
Vascular changes		
Telangiectasia	Ectatic vessels often with atrophic walls	Acutely, UV exposure stimulates angiogenesis through vascular endothelial growth factor upregulation via MEK-ERK activation and thrombospondim-1 downregulation via P13K-Akt activation in human epidermis, although with chronic exposure blood vessels may be decreased in UV-damaged skin
Senile purpura	Extravasated erythrocytes and increased perivascular inflammation	Blood vessel fragility by decreased collagen and elastic fibers

Table 1. Clinical and histological features of photoaged skin and related molecular mechanisms.

4.2. Matrix metalloproteinases and signal transduction pathways

Matrix metalloproteinases (MMPs) are an important family of zinc-containing proteinases that have the capacity to degrade most of the extracellular matrix proteins that comprise the structure of the skin dermal connective tissue [24, 25]. During the past 20 years, a remarkable amount of research has been conducted into both skin aging and MMPs, which can play a significant role in the aging process in the skin. In 1996, Fisher et al. [26] observed that MMP expression was induced and activated after UVB irradiation of the human skin. The molecular model proposed by Fisher et al. suggests that UV radiation can activate various growth factor and cytokine receptors on the cell surface and stimulate mitogen-activated protein kinase (MAPK) signal transduction, which then upregulates transcription factors activator protein-1 (AP-1) composed of c-Jun and c-Fos proteins, and nuclear factor kappa B (NF-κB) in the nucleus. The induction of AP-1 elevates MMP expression, including MMP-1 (collagenase), MMP-3 (stromelysin-1), and MMP-9 (92 kDa gelatinase), and results in the degradation of extracellular matrix components in human skin *in vivo* [1, 27]. This degradation results in accumulation of fragmented, disorganized collagen fibrils, and these damaged collagen products downregulate new collagen synthesis, which suggests that collagen synthesis is negatively regulated by collagen breakdown [28, 29]. The combined actions of MMP-1, MMP-3, and MMP-9 degrade most of type I and III dermal collagen. Furthermore, AP-1 inhibits procollagen biosynthesis by suppressing gene expression of type I and III procollagen in the dermis, which results in a reduced collagen content [25]. The data indicate that epidermal keratinocytes are a major cellular source of MMPs that are produced in response to exposure of human skin to solar UV irradiation. However, dermal cells may also play a role in epidermal production of MMPs, through indirect paracrine mechanisms, by release of growth factors or cytokines, which in turn modulate MMP production by epidermal keratinocytes.

4.3. Oxidative stress

Free radicals are considered the major contributors to the aging process of skin through the accumulation of ROS. The free radical theory postulates that extremely reactive chemical molecules are a major cause of the aging process [30]. The status of oxidant–antioxidant imbalance is referred to as oxidative stress. Oxidative stress occurring in cells can lead to the oxidation of cell membrane phospholipids, which results in the distortion of the transmembrane signaling pathway [31]. Generally, increased ROS production leads to the activation of MAPK. MAPK induces AP-1, which consequently increases the expression of MMPs, resulting in a decrease of collagen in aged skin [32]. Oxidative stress also contributes to the increased oxidation of macromolecules, such as cellular lipids, proteins, and DNA, which causes cellular dysfunction with age. Age-related accumulation of damaged, oxidized, and aggregated altered proteins might lead to aging [31, 33]. Oxidative protein damage is the most common molecular sign of aging and is observed in photodamaged skin through ROS-mediated protein damage in the upper dermis [33]. Cellular accumulation of lipofuscin, a large protein–lipid aggregate, gradually increases with age, eventually inhibiting proteasome function [31]. Disruption of the epidermal calcium gradient is observed in aged skin because of changes in the composition of the cornified envelope, which results in reduced epidermal barrier function [31].

4.4. Vascular alterations

Human skin is affected by various environmental conditions such as solar UV radiation, infrared (IR) radiation, and heat, and these stimuli can contribute to skin angiogenesis. Interestingly, although the exposure of acute UV radiation stimulates skin angiogenesis, blood vessels of skin are decreased in chronically photodamaged skin. These differential effects of acute and chronic UV radiation on skin angiogenesis remain unknown. Acute and chronic UV irradiation of skin influences angiogenesis. UV irradiation induces angiogenesis via the upregulation of vascular endothelial growth factor and inhibition of thrombospondin-1, a potent inhibitor of angiogenesis [34].

4.5. Cytokines in skin aging

Cytokines play a central role in the visible clinical signs of aging [35]. Tumor necrosis factor α (TNF-α), which has a key role in proinflammatory process in skin, inhibits collagen synthesis and induces the production of MMP-9 [35, 36]. 3-Deoxysappanchalcone inhibits MMP-9 expression through the suppression of AP-1 and NF-κB in human skin keratinocytes [36]. Furthermore, high concentrations of TNF-α are correlated with a decrease of collagen production via induction of collagenase activity in fibroblasts [37]. Levels of interleukin (IL)-1 and

IL-18 increase with age and promote skin inflammation, which causes age-related processes [38]. UV radiation exposure stimulated IL-1 receptor antagonist (IL-1ra), a competitive inhibitor of IL-1, although IL-1ra production in the skin decreased with age. IL-1ra has a regulatory role in the IL-1 related proinflammatory response, and may play a role in the regulation of IL-1-induced inflammatory responses, and maintain an appropriate balance between IL-1 and IL-1ra [38]. IL-18, an IL-1 superfamily cytokine, is a pleiotropic immune regulator that functions as an angiogenic mediator in inflammation [39]. IL-18 has been implicated as a strong proinflammatory mediator in the pathogenesis of age-related diseases by inducing interferon-γ [39]. In addition, another proinflammatory cytokine, IL-6, increases after menopause and is associated with the formation of skin wrinkles [40]. IL-6 levels are upregulated on exposure to UV radiation [41]. Increased levels of cysteine-rich protein 61 (CCN1) are observed in dermal fibroblasts with age, and CCN1 contributes to the skin connective tissue aging by collagen reduction and degradation in aged human skin *in vivo* [42]. Furthermore, CCN1 induced age-associated secretory proteins, including various proinflammatory cytokines and MMPs, which results in aging of connective tissue [42].

4.6. Other environmental stressors in skin aging

4.6.1. Tobacco smoke

Like UV radiation exposure, smoking can result in extrinsic skin aging. Findings from large epidemiological studies imply that there is a link between tobacco smoking and premature skin aging [43–45]. Skin damage from long-term smoking can result in a "smoker's face" and can cause facial skin to appear grayish and lines to develop around the eyes and mouth, through damage to collagen fibers and elastin in the dermis [46]. Significantly increased levels of MMP-1 mRNA are observed in the dermal connective tissue of smokers compared with nonsmokers [47]. Increased MMP-1 leads to the degradation of collagen and elastic fibers, which are major extracellular matrix proteins in the dermis. To confirm the pathogenic role of tobacco in skin aging, Morita et al. [46] showed that topical application of water-soluble tobacco smoke extract to the backs of mice led to a loss of collagen bundles and a concomitant increase of damaged collagen in the upper dermis, which mimicked age-related skin. Furthermore, several *in vitro* studies provided possible pathomechanisms for the association between tobacco smoke extract and skin aging. Tobacco smoke extract reduces procollagen types I and III and induced the production of MMP-1 and 3, which degrades extracellular matrix proteins, and also results in abnormal regulation of extracellular matrix deposition in human cultured skin fibroblasts [48]. Tobacco smoke extract also inhibited cellular responsiveness to transforming growth factor-β (TGF-β), a key mediator of collagen synthesis through the induction of a nonfunctional form of TGF-β, and downregulation of the TGF-β receptor in supernatants of cultured skin fibroblasts, leading to decreased synthesis of extracellular matrix [49]. Moreover, tobacco smoke is a major source of polycyclic aromatic hydrocarbon exposure in humans. In this regard, it has been shown that tobacco smoke extract induced MMP-1 expression via activation of the aryl hydrocarbon receptor (AhR) signaling pathway in human fibroblasts and keratinocytes [50].

4.6.2. *Infrared radiation and heat*

Heat energy may be transmitted by IR radiation, which increases skin temperature. Lee et al. [51] found that the temperature of human skin can increase to about 40°C under IR irradiation following the conversion of absorbed IR radiation into heat energy. Chronic exposure of skin to heat may cause premature skin aging, just like UV radiation. The expression of MMP-1 and MMP-3 is induced by heat shock in cultured normal human skin fibroblasts through ERK and JNK activation [52]. Decreased type I procollagen levels and increased MMP-1 expression were observed in human skin exposed to IR radiation, which suggests that chronic IR irradiation can cause skin wrinkling [53]. MMP-12, which is the most active MMP against elastic fiber network in human skin, was induced after heat treatment *in vivo* and thereby contributed to the development of solar elastosis in photoaged skin, thereby contributing to premature skin aging [54]. IR irradiation induces an angiogenic switch by the upregulation of vascular endothelial growth factor and downregulation of thrombospondin-2, which leads to angiogenesis and inflammation in human skin *in vivo* [55].

4.6.3. *Environmental pollutants*

Exposure to outdoor air pollution from traffic and industry is associated with an increased risk of signs of extrinsic skin aging, in particular pigmented spots and wrinkles in white women of European ancestry [56]. Polycyclic aromatic hydrocarbons are the major participants and trigger the AhR signaling pathway, because their lipophilicity enables them to penetrate the skin easily. Activation of the AhR pathway increases MMP-1 expression in the normal human keratinocytes [57]. In addition, AhR signaling pathway could contribute to the modulate melanogenesis by upregulating tyrosinase enzyme activity [58]. These findings suggest that polycyclic aromatic hydrocarbon-induced AhR activation may play a significant role in the formation of dark pigmentation and coarse wrinkles, which are clinical hallmarks of extrinsic aging. Indoor air pollution released by the combustion of solid fuels for heating is a major environmental and public health challenge in developing countries [59]. Recently, Li et al. [60] reported that indoor air pollution from cooking with solid fuels was significantly associated with 5–8% deeper facial wrinkles and folds and an increased risk of developing fine wrinkles on the dorsum of hands in Chinese women. It is thus likely that exposure to indoor combustion of solid fuels might induce the same molecular pathways in skin cells as outdoor pollution and thereby cause wrinkle formation.

5. Molecular aspects of antiaging treatments

5.1. Topical retinoids

Topical retinoids (vitamin A derivatives, also known as retinol) are the main stay of treatment of patients gradually photoaging [61]. Tretinoin and tazarotene are the only two topical retinoids that are currently U.S. Food and Drug Administration (FDA) approved for the treatment of photoaging. The detailed mechanism of action of retinoids has been elucidated.

They bind to and activate the retinoic acid receptors (RARs), which are present in a nuclear and work in pairs. These nuclear receptors have two binding sites, which is one for the ligands (retinoid), and one for specific DNA sequences of a target gene. In the presence of the ligands, those heterodimers can recognize a DNA sequence and regulate transcription. Their signal transduction is believed to be implicated in the synthesis of procollagen, thus increasing the formation of type I and III collagen, and inhibiting MMPs [1, 26]. Although the precise mechanisms are unknown, the induction of dermal collagen appears to be a crucial factor. Retinoic acid stimulated production of type VII collagen (anchoring fibrils) and type I collagen [4]. Clinically, retinoids reduce the appearance of fine lines, improve skin texture, correct tone and elasticity, and slow the progression of photoaging. The clinical improvements of topical retinoid therapy are typically seen after several weeks of therapy [62, 63]. A 24-month, double-blind, vehicle-controlled, multicenter study of tretinoin cream versus vehicle in the treatment of photoaged facial skin was conducted. Topical administration of tretinoin cream for 24 months has proved to be effective in treating clinical signs including fine wrinkling at 2 months, hyperpigmentation at 4 months, coarse wrinkling at 1 month, and sallowness at 4 months [64]. In addition to these clinical benefits, the following histopathological effects are well documented: epidermal hyperplasia and thickening, a decrease of epidermal melanin content, an increase of collagen synthesis, and a decrease of dermal collagen breakdown by inhibiting MMPs and a decrease of p53 expression [65]. Topical retinoids may cause an irritant reaction such as erythema, scaling, burning sensation, and dermatitis, and these reactions cause to decrease patient compliance. Therefore, retinoids should be initiated at the lowest effective dose to minimize adverse reactions [66]. Although tazarotene is the only topical retinoid with a category X designation, topical retinoids are not recommended during pregnancy or lactation [67].

5.2. Cosmeceuticals

Cosmeceuticals encompass a heterogeneous category of nonprescription topical products, including antioxidants, vitamins, hydroxy acids, and plant extracts [68]. Cosmeceuticals are marketed to the consumer based on the claims of their antiaging effects. Although some products may have scientific rationale and produce visible results in the treatment of photoaging, they are not classified as drugs. Most have not been studied thoroughly, especially on human skin, and these products are not subject to the rigorous testing or regulation by agencies such as the FDA. However, the most cosmeceuticals serve a role in keeping the skin moisturized, maintain the homeostasis of the skin, and many are combined with a topical retinol to enhance their antiaging benefits. As mentioned above, UV and IR irradiation of skin leads to free radical formation. It has been hypothesized that antioxidants scavenge these free radicals and thus protect cells from damage. The antioxidants include coenzyme Q, lipoic acid, vitamin C, and vitamin E [69–71]. Among the many cosmeceuticals, there is increasing interest in botanical antioxidants. Representatively, green tea polyphenols (GTPs) have gained attention because of their potent antioxidant activities. In animal models, UV radiation-induced cutaneous edema and cyclooxygenase activity could be significantly inhibited by feeding GTPs to the animals. After topical application of creams containing GTPs, GTPs on mouse skin decreased the UV-induced hyperplasia, edema, and myeloperoxidase activity. Epigallocatechin-3-gallate (EGCG), which is a polyphenolic constituent of GTP, has been reported to have the inhibitory effect on the expression and activity of MMPs and leukocyte elastase, which has an important role in tumor invasion and metastasis. In addition, GTPs have been shown to decrease the levels of oxidative stress, prevent UV radiation-induced DNA damage, their potential immunosuppressive effects, and skin cancers [72, 73]. Like GTPs, other botanic extracts have been described to contain potent antioxidant components, including curcumin (turmeric), silymarin (milk thistle), apigenin, resveratrol (red grape), and genistein (soy bean) [74]. In fact, recently, it has been demonstrated that these components can inhibit the inflammatory response by downregulation of various proinflammatory mediators, inhibition of activated immune cells, or inhibiting inducible nitric oxide synthase (iNOS) and cyclooxygenase-2 (COX-2) via its inhibitory effects on NF-κB or AP-1 [75]. Further investigations are needed to focus on the potential application of cosmeceuticals and determine how they can contribute to improvements in skin aging at the maximum.

5.3. Cytokines and growth factors

Cytokines play a crucial role in the development of clinical features of skin aging. Numerous proinflammatory cytokines including TNF-α, IL-1, and IL-18 can affect the aging process by triggering collagen breakdown via upregulation of MMP-9. These inflammatory cytokines can lower the skin immunity and thus increases the risk of skin infections in old age [35]. Many growth factors are involved in wound healing and have the ability to increase fibroblast and keratinocyte proliferation within the dermis, thus inducing extracellular matrix formation [76]. Growth factors are produced and secreted by many skin cell types, including fibroblasts, keratinocytes, and melanocytes. These secreted growth factors are those that regulate the immune system, also known as cytokines [77, 78]. It is important to combine growth factors and cytokines (referred to collectively as GFs) because they work together and regulate each other via inter- and intracellular signaling pathways. The defined role of GFs in healing of skin wounds allows a parallel model to be developed for the role of GFs in skin rejuvenation. Like the skin wound-healing process, topical and injectable GFs have the potential to modify complex cellular network leading to the increase of collagen synthesis and decrease of collagen degradation. Therefore, they have emerged as an intriguing therapeutic modality to address skin aging through the stimulation of cell regeneration [79, 80]. In fact, topical GFs can cross the skin barrier and bind to cell surface receptors, which trigger a signaling cascade and lead to stimulate keratinocyte proliferation [81]. However, a limited number of controlled studies demonstrate that topically applied GFs can stimulate collagen synthesis and epidermal thickening, which is associated with clinical improvement in signs of photoaging. Because the use of GFs is still in an early stage, continued study to determine their efficacy is needed.

5.4. Neurotoxins and dermal fillers

Over the past 10 years, the use of botulinum toxin and dermal fillers for aesthetic purposes has risen sharply. Botulinum toxin is an injectable neuromodulator used to reduce fine lines and wrinkles. The toxin functions by inhibiting acetylcholine release at the neuromuscular junction, resulting in flaccid paralysis of targeted muscles [82]. It has been demonstrated that botulinum toxin decreased both collagen synthesis and the expression of MMP-9 in human dermal fibroblasts *in vitro*, leading to decreases collagen degradation [83]. Furthermore, botulinum toxin can also stimulate the expression of type I collagen in human dermal fibroblasts, suggesting that botulinum toxin can stimulate remodeling of ECM, an essential for the rejuvenation of skin aging [83].

Dermal filler injections are used to improve coarse wrinkles and gradual loss of tissue volume [84]. Regardless of trade name, products with smaller particles (softer consistency) are the most useful for superficial injection to address fine lines, whereas larger particle (stiffer) hyaluronic fillers (HA fillers) are the best suited for deeper injection to treat volume loss and deep rhytids [85]. In general, superficial "fine-line" products last approximately 6 months or more, whereas larger particle products last for 6–12 months. In recent years, combination treatment with botulinum toxin and fillers was recommended to achieve superior clinical outcomes and greater patient satisfaction [86, 87].

Several studies demonstrated that fibroblasts in aged skin could be "rejuvenated" by enhancing structural support and mechanical force by injection of dermal filler, cross-linked hyaluronic acid, into the skin [88]. In addition, injection of dermal HA filler can stimulate fibroblasts to produce type I collagen associated with increase in mechanical forces. Enhanced mechanical support of the ECM also stimulates the fibroblast, endothelial cells, and keratinocytes proliferation, resulting in increase of vasculature and epidermal thickness mediated by upregulation of TGF-β receptor and various growth factors. Consistent with these observations in human skin, injection of dermal filler into dermal equivalent cultures *in vitro* induces elongation of fibroblasts and type I collagen synthesis by enhancing structural support of the ECM [88].

5.5. Lasers and other novel devices

Laser resurfacing is a skin rejuvenation technology developed to target the cutaneous signs of photodamage. Lasers and other light source procedures are divided into ablative and nonablative resurfacing. Laser procedures are based on the theory of selective photothermolysis [89]. Ablative lasers were first used in the 1980s and markedly improved rhytids, dyspigmentation, skin laxity, and other signs of photoaging by inducing dermal collagen remodeling. The traditional ablative lasers consisted of the 10,600-nm CO_2 and 2940-nm erbium-doped yttrium aluminum garnet (Er:YAG) lasers. Ablative laser resurfacing employs CO_2 and Er:YAG lasers, which both target water as their chromophore. CO_2 lasers emit light at 10,600 nm in the far-IR electromagnetic spectrum [90, 91]. Er:YAG lasers, introduced in 1996, emit light at 2940 nm, closer to the absorption peak of water, which results in very superficial absorption of laser light [92]. When compared with a CO_2 laser, the absorption coefficient for the Er:YAG laser is 16 times higher [93]. Ablative laser resurfacing provides significant improvement of photodamaged skin, photoinduced rhytids, dyschromias, and scars. However, because of the relatively high risk of adverse effects and long recovery period, fractional ablative and other nonablative lasers have since been developed. Nonablative lasers have been developed as an alternative to traditional ablative resurfacing with the aim to comply with patients' new demands for short healing time and reduced discomfort and are widely used for dermal collagen remodeling [94, 95]. Long-pulsed 1064-nm neodymium-doped (Nd): YAG laser treatment increased dermal collagen and decreased the expression of MMP-1 associated with the increased expression of TGF-β [96]. Fractional radiofrequency therapy is a novel, noninvasive method of tissue tightening. Radiowave energy is delivered deep into the skin, which causes water in the skin cells to heat up, stimulating the production of heat-shock proteins and promoting the wound-healing response [97]. Side effects including dyspigmentation, keloids, or thermal injury can occur and need to be considered. Therefore, in managing photoaging, treatments should be tailored to target the specific clinical features in different skin types and ethnic origin of the patients, and sufficient epidermal cooling after the treatment is required [98].

Acknowledgements

This work was supported by the Basic Science Research program through the National Research Foundation of Korea (NRF), which is funded by the Ministry of Education, Science and Technology (2015R1C1A2A01055073).

Author details

Miri Kim and Hyun Jeong Park*

*Address all correspondence to: hjpark@catholic.ac.kr

Department of Dermatology, Yeouido St. Mary's Hospital, The Catholic University of Korea, Seoul, Korea

References

[1] Fisher, G.J., et al., *Mechanisms of photoaging and chronological skin aging*. Arch Dermatol, 2002. 138(11): pp. 1462–70.

[2] Murakami, H., et al., *Importance of amino acid composition to improve skin collagen protein synthesis rates in UV-irradiated mice*. Amino Acids, 2012. 42(6): pp. 2481–9.

[3] Kang, S., G.J. Fisher, and J.J. Voorhees, *Photoaging: pathogenesis, prevention, and treatment*. Clin Geriatr Med, 2001. 17(4): pp. 643–59, v-vi.

[4] Han, A., A.L. Chien, and S. Kang, *Photoaging*. Dermatol Clin, 2014. 32(3): pp. 291–9, vii.

[5] Lavker, R.M., *Structural alterations in exposed and unexposed aged skin*. J Investig Dermatol, 1979. 73(1): pp. 59–66.

[6] Yaar, M. and B.A. Gilchrest, *Photoageing: mechanism, prevention and therapy*. Br J Dermatol, 2007. 157(5): pp. 874–87.

[7] Gilchrest, B.A., F.B. Blog, and G. Szabo, *Effects of aging and chronic sun exposure on melanocytes in human skin*. J Investig Dermatol, 1979. 73(2): pp. 141–3.

[8] Varani, J., et al., *Vascular tube formation on matrix metalloproteinase-1-damaged collagen*. Br J Cancer, 2008. 98(10): pp. 1646–52.

[9] Braverman, I.M. and E. Fonferko, *Studies in cutaneous aging: I. The elastic fiber network*. J Investig Dermatol, 1982. 78(5): pp. 434–43.

[10] Zouboulis Ch, C., *[Intrinsic skin aging. A critical appraisal of the role of hormones]*. Hautarzt, 2003. 54(9): pp. 825–32.

[11] Kurban, R.S. and J. Bhawan, *Histologic changes in skin associated with aging*. J Dermatol Surg Oncol, 1990. 16(10): pp. 908–14.

[12] Bhawan, J., et al., *Photoaging versus intrinsic aging: a morphologic assessment of facial skin*. J Cutan Pathol, 1995. 22(2): pp. 154–9.

[13] Eller, M.S., M. Yaar, and B.A. Gilchrest, *DNA damage and melanogenesis*. Nature, 1994. 372(6505): pp. 413–4.

[14] Schwarz, T., *Photoimmunosuppression*. Photodermatol Photoimmunol Photomed, 2002. 18(3): pp. 141–5.

[15] Bosset, S., et al., *Photoageing shows histological features of chronic skin inflammation without clinical and molecular abnormalities*. Br J Dermatol, 2003. 149(4): pp. 826–35.

[16] Varani, J., et al., *Vitamin A antagonizes decreased cell growth and elevated collagen-degrading matrix metalloproteinases and stimulates collagen accumulation in naturally aged human skin*. J Investig Dermatol, 2000. 114(3): pp. 480–6.

[17] Tsuji, T., *Loss of dermal elastic tissue in solar elastosis*. Arch Dermatol, 1980. 116(4): pp. 474–5.

[18] Sellheyer, K., *Pathogenesis of solar elastosis: synthesis or degradation?* J Cutan Pathol, 2003. 30(2): pp. 123–7.

[19] Sugimoto, M., R. Yamashita, and M. Ueda, *Telomere length of the skin in association with chronological aging and photoaging*. J Dermatol Sci, 2006. 43(1): pp. 43–7.

[20] Aubert, G. and P.M. Lansdorp, *Telomeres and aging*. Physiol Rev, 2008. 88(2): pp. 557–79.

[21] Buckingham, E.M. and A.J. Klingelhutz, *The role of telomeres in the ageing of human skin*. Exp Dermatol, 2011. 20(4): pp. 297–302.

[22] Cong, Y.S., W.E. Wright, and J.W. Shay, *Human telomerase and its regulation*. Microbiol Mol Biol Rev, 2002. 66(3): pp. 407–25, table of contents.

[23] Oikawa, S., S. Tada-Oikawa, and S. Kawanishi, *Site-specific DNA damage at the GGG sequence by UVA involves acceleration of telomere shortening*. Biochemistry, 2001. 40(15): pp. 4763–8.

[24] Nelson, A.R., et al., *Matrix metalloproteinases: biologic activity and clinical implications*. J Clin Oncol, 2000. 18(5): pp. 1135–49.

[25] Sternlicht, M.D. and Z. Werb, *How matrix metalloproteinases regulate cell behavior*. Annu Rev Cell Dev Biol, 2001. 17: pp. 463–516.

[26] Fisher, G.J., et al., *Molecular basis of sun-induced premature skin ageing and retinoid antagonism*. Nature, 1996. 379(6563): pp. 335–9.

[27] Fisher, G.J., et al., *Retinoic acid inhibits induction of c-Jun protein by ultraviolet radiation that occurs subsequent to activation of mitogen-activated protein kinase pathways in human skin in vivo*. J Clin Investig, 1998. 101(6): pp. 1432–40.

[28] Fligiel, S.E., et al., *Collagen degradation in aged/photodamaged skin in vivo and after exposure to matrix metalloproteinase-1 in vitro*. J Investig Dermatol, 2003. 120(5): pp. 842–8.

[29] Quan, T., et al., *Matrix-degrading metalloproteinases in photoaging*. J Investig Dermatol Symp Proc, 2009. 14(1): pp. 20–4.

[30] Piotrowska, A. and E. Bartnik, *[The role of reactive oxygen species and mitochondria in aging]*. Postepy Biochem, 2014. 60(2): pp. 240–7.

[31] Rinnerthaler, M., et al., *Oxidative stress in aging human skin*. Biomolecules, 2015. 5(2): pp. 545–89.

[32] Son, Y., et al., *Mitogen-activated protein kinases and reactive oxygen species: how can ROS activate MAPK pathways?* J Signal Transduct, 2011. 2011: pp. 792639.

[33] Hipkiss, A.R., *Accumulation of altered proteins and ageing: causes and effects*. Exp Gerontol, 2006. 41(5): pp. 464–73.

[34] Chung, J.H. and H.C. Eun, *Angiogenesis in skin aging and photoaging*. J Dermatol, 2007. 34(9): pp. 593–600.

[35] Borg, M., et al., *The role of cytokines in skin aging*. Climacteric, 2013. 16(5): pp. 514–21.

[36] Youn, U.J., et al., *3-Deoxysappanchalcone inhibits tumor necrosis factor-alpha-induced matrix metalloproteinase-9 expression in human keratinocytes through activated protein-1 inhibition and nuclear factor-kappa B DNA binding activity*. Biol Pharm Bull, 2011. 34(6): pp. 890–3.

[37] Chou, D.H., W. Lee, and C.A. McCulloch, *TNF-alpha inactivation of collagen receptors: implications for fibroblast function and fibrosis*. J Immunol, 1996. 156(11): pp. 4354–62.

[38] Hirao, T., et al., *Elevation of interleukin 1 receptor antagonist in the stratum corneum of sun-exposed and ultraviolet B-irradiated human skin*. J Investig Dermatol, 1996. 106(5): pp. 1102–7.

[39] Lee, J.H., D.H. Cho, and H.J. Park, *IL-18 and cutaneous inflammatory diseases*. Int J Mol Sci, 2015. 16(12): pp. 29357–69.

[40] Kim, O.Y., et al., *Effects of aging and menopause on serum interleukin-6 levels and peripheral blood mononuclear cell cytokine production in healthy nonobese women*. Age (Dordr), 2012. 34(2): pp. 415–25.

[41] Omoigui, S., *The Interleukin-6 inflammation pathway from cholesterol to aging—role of statins, bisphosphonates and plant polyphenols in aging and age-related diseases*. Immun Ageing, 2007. 4: p. 1.

[42] Quan, T., et al., *CCN1 contributes to skin connective tissue aging by inducing age-associated secretory phenotype in human skin dermal fibroblasts*. J Cell Commun Signal, 2011. 5(3): pp. 201–7.

[43] Kadunce, D.P., et al., *Cigarette smoking: risk factor for premature facial wrinkling*. Ann Intern Med, 1991. 114(10): pp. 840–4.

[44] Ernster, V.L., et al., *Facial wrinkling in men and women, by smoking status*. Am J Public Health, 1995. 85(1): pp. 78–82.

[45] Morita, A., *Tobacco smoke causes premature skin aging*. J Dermatol Sci, 2007. 48(3): pp. 169–75.

[46] Morita, A., et al., *Molecular basis of tobacco smoke-induced premature skin aging*. J Investig Dermatol Symp Proc, 2009. 14(1): pp. 53–5.

[47] Lahmann, C., et al., *Matrix metalloproteinase-1 and skin ageing in smokers*. Lancet, 2001. 357(9260): pp. 935–6.

[48] Yin, L., A. Morita, and T. Tsuji, *Alterations of extracellular matrix induced by tobacco smoke extract*. Arch Dermatol Res, 2000. 292(4): pp. 188–94.

[49] Yin, L., A. Morita, and T. Tsuji, *Tobacco smoke extract induces age-related changes due to modulation of TGF-beta*. Exp Dermatol, 2003. 12 Suppl 2: pp. 51–6.

[50] Ono, Y., et al., *Role of the aryl hydrocarbon receptor in tobacco smoke extract-induced matrix metalloproteinase-1 expression*. Exp Dermatol, 2013. 22(5): pp. 349–53.

[51] Lee, H.S., et al., *Minimal heating dose: a novel biological unit to measure infrared irradiation*. Photodermatol Photoimmunol Photomed, 2006. 22(3): pp. 148–52.

[52] Park, C.H., et al., *Heat shock-induced matrix metalloproteinase (MMP) 1 and MMP-3 are mediated through ERK and JNK activation and via an autocrine interleukin-6 loop*. J Investig Dermatol, 2004. 123(6): pp. 1012–9.

[53] Kim, M.S., et al., *Regulation of type I procollagen and MMP-1 expression after single or repeated exposure to infrared radiation in human skin*. Mech Ageing Dev, 2006. 127(12): pp. 875–82.

[54] Chen, Z., et al., *Heat modulation of tropoelastin, fibrillin-1, and matrix metalloproteinase-12 in human skin in vivo.* J Investig Dermatol, 2005. 124(1): pp. 70–8.

[55] Kim, M.S., et al., *Infrared exposure induces an angiogenic switch in human skin that is partially mediated by heat.* Br J Dermatol, 2006. 155(6): pp. 1131–8.

[56] Vierkotter, A., et al., *Airborne particle exposure and extrinsic skin aging.* J Investig Dermatol, 2010. 130(12): pp. 2719–26.

[57] Murphy, K.A., et al., *Interaction between the aryl hydrocarbon receptor and retinoic acid pathways increases matrix metalloproteinase-1 expression in keratinocytes.* J Biol Chem, 2004. 279(24): pp. 25284–93.

[58] Luecke, S., et al., *The aryl hydrocarbon receptor (AHR), a novel regulator of human melanogenesis.* Pigment Cell Melanoma Res, 2010. 23(6): pp. 828–33.

[59] Bruce, N., R. Perez-Padilla, and R. Albalak, *Indoor air pollution in developing countries: a major environmental and public health challenge.* Bull World Health Organ, 2000. 78(9): pp. 1078–92.

[60] Li, M., et al., *Epidemiological evidence that indoor air pollution from cooking with solid fuels accelerates skin aging in Chinese women.* J Dermatol Sci, 2015. 79(2): pp. 148–54.

[61] Kligman, A.M., et al., *Topical tretinoin for photoaged skin.* J Am Acad Dermatol, 1986. 15(4 Pt 2): pp. 836–59.

[62] Griffiths, C.E., et al., *Two concentrations of topical tretinoin (retinoic acid) cause similar improvement of photoaging but different degrees of irritation. A double-blind, vehicle-controlled comparison of 0.1% and 0.025% tretinoin creams.* Arch Dermatol, 1995. 131(9): pp. 1037–44.

[63] Kang, S., et al., *Tazarotene cream for the treatment of facial photodamage: a multicenter, investigator-masked, randomized, vehicle-controlled, parallel comparison of 0.01%, 0.025%, 0.05%, and 0.1% tazarotene creams with 0.05% tretinoin emollient cream applied once daily for 24 weeks.* Arch Dermatol, 2001. 137(12): pp. 1597–604.

[64] Berger, R., et al., *A double-blinded, randomized, vehicle-controlled, multicenter, parallel-group study to assess the safety and efficacy of tretinoin gel microsphere 0.04% in the treatment of acne vulgaris in adults.* Cutis, 2007. 80(2): pp. 152–7.

[65] Griffiths, C.E., et al., *Treatment of photoaged skin with a cream containing 0.05% isotretinoin and sunscreens.* J Dermatol Treat, 2005. 16(2): pp. 79–86.

[66] Samuel, M., et al., *Interventions for photodamaged skin.* Cochrane Database Syst Rev, 2005(1): p. CD001782.

[67] Antoniou, C., et al., *Photoaging: prevention and topical treatments.* Am J Clin Dermatol, 2010. 11(2): pp. 95–102.

[68] Draelos, Z.D., *The art and science of new advances in cosmeceuticals*. Clin Plast Surg, 2011. 38(3): pp. 397–407, vi.

[69] Geesin, J.C., et al., *Ascorbic acid specifically increases type I and type III procollagen messenger RNA levels in human skin fibroblast*. J Investig Dermatol, 1988. 90(4): pp. 420–4.

[70] Keller, K.L. and N.A. Fenske, *Uses of vitamins A, C, and E and related compounds in dermatology: a review*. J Am Acad Dermatol, 1998. 39(4 Pt 1): pp. 611–25.

[71] Matsugo, S., T. Bito, and T. Konishi, *Photochemical stability of lipoic acid and its impact on skin ageing*. Free Radic Res, 2011. 45(8): pp. 918–24.

[72] Roh, E., et al., *Molecular mechanisms of green tea polyphenols with protective effects against skin photoaging*. Crit Rev Food Sci Nutr, 2015: p. 0.

[73] Vayalil, P.K., et al., *Green tea polyphenols prevent ultraviolet light-induced oxidative damage and matrix metalloproteinases expression in mouse skin*. J Investig Dermatol, 2004. 122(6): pp. 1480–7.

[74] Poljsak, B., R. Dahmane, and A. Godic, *Skin and antioxidants*. J Cosmet Laser Ther, 2013. 15(2): pp. 107–13.

[75] de la Lastra, C.A. and I. Villegas, *Resveratrol as an anti-inflammatory and anti-aging agent: mechanisms and clinical implications*. Mol Nutr Food Res, 2005. 49(5): pp. 405–30.

[76] Bonin-Debs, A.L., et al., *Development of secreted proteins as biotherapeutic agents*. Expert Opin Biol Ther, 2004. 4(4): pp. 551–8.

[77] Martin, P., *Wound healing–aiming for perfect skin regeneration*. Science, 1997. 276(5309): pp. 75–81.

[78] Moulin, V., *Growth factors in skin wound healing*. Eur J Cell Biol, 1995. 68(1): pp. 1–7.

[79] Araki, J., et al., *Optimized preparation method of platelet-concentrated plasma and noncoagulating platelet-derived factor concentrates: maximization of platelet concentration and removal of fibrinogen*. Tissue Eng Part C Methods, 2012. 18(3): pp. 176–85.

[80] Sundaram, H., et al., *Topically applied physiologically balanced growth factors: a new paradigm of skin rejuvenation*. J Drugs Dermatol, 2009. 8(5 Suppl Skin Rejuenation): pp. 4–13.

[81] Fabi, S. and H. Sundaram, *The potential of topical and injectable growth factors and cytokines for skin rejuvenation*. Facial Plast Surg, 2014. 30(2): pp. 157–71.

[82] Carruthers, J. and A. Carruthers, *The evolution of botulinum neurotoxin type A for cosmetic applications*. J Cosmet Laser Ther, 2007. 9(3): pp. 186–92.

[83] Oh, S.H., et al., *The potential effect of botulinum toxin type A on human dermal fibroblasts: an in vitro study*. Dermatol Surg, 2012. 38(10): pp. 1689–94.

[84] Klein, A.W., *Techniques for soft tissue augmentation: an 'a to z'*. Am J Clin Dermatol, 2006. 7(2): pp. 107–20.

[85] De Boulle, K., *Management of complications after implantation of fillers*. J Cosmet Dermatol, 2004. 3(1): pp. 2–15.

[86] Patel, M.P., M. Talmor, and W.B. Nolan, *Botox and collagen for glabellar furrows: advantages of combination therapy*. Ann Plast Surg, 2004. 52(5): pp. 442–7; discussion 447.

[87] Coleman, K.R. and J. Carruthers, *Combination therapy with BOTOX and fillers: the new rejuvnation paradigm*. Dermatol Ther, 2006. 19(3): pp. 177–88.

[88] Quan, T., et al., *Enhancing structural support of the dermal microenvironment activates fibroblasts, endothelial cells, and keratinocytes in aged human skin in vivo*. J Investig Dermatol, 2013. 133(3): pp. 658–67.

[89] Anderson, R.R. and J.A. Parrish, *Selective photothermolysis: precise microsurgery by selective absorption of pulsed radiation*. Science, 1983. 220(4596): pp. 524–7.

[90] Ratner, D., et al., *Cutaneous laser resurfacing*. J Am Acad Dermatol, 1999. 41(3 Pt 1): pp. 365–89; quiz 390–2.

[91] Walsh, J.T., Jr., et al., *Pulsed CO2 laser tissue ablation: effect of tissue type and pulse duration on thermal damage*. Lasers Surg Med, 1988. 8(2): pp. 108–18.

[92] Zachary, C.B., *Modulating the Er:YAG laser*. Lasers Surg Med, 2000. 26(2): pp. 223–6.

[93] Alster, T.S., C.A. Nanni, and C.M. Williams, *Comparison of four carbon dioxide resurfacing lasers. A clinical and histopathologic evaluation*. Dermatol Surg, 1999. 25(3): pp. 153–8; discussion 159.

[94] Alam, M. and J.S. Dover, *Nonablative laser and light therapy: an approach to patient and device selection*. Skin Therapy Lett, 2003. 8(4): pp. 4–7.

[95] Zelickson, B.D., et al., *Pulsed dye laser therapy for sun damaged skin*. Lasers Surg Med, 1999. 25(3): pp. 229–36.

[96] Lee, Y.B., et al., *Effects of long-pulsed 1,064-nm neodymium-doped yttrium aluminum garnet laser on dermal collagen remodeling in hairless mice*. Dermatol Surg, 2012. 38(7 Pt 1): pp. 985–92.

[97] Bodendorf, M.O., et al., *Fractional laser skin therapy*. J Dtsch Dermatol Ges, 2009. 7(4): pp. 301–8.

[98] Munavalli, G.S., R.A. Weiss, and R.M. Halder, *Photoaging and nonablative photorejuvenation in ethnic skin*. Dermatol Surg, 2005. 31(9 Pt 2): pp. 1250–60; discussion 1261.

Chapter 5

The Rejuvenation of the Immune System: Physiological, Cellular, and Molecular Mechanisms

Iryna Pishel and Gennadij Butenko

Additional information is available at the end of the chapter

http://dx.doi.org/10.5772/64046

Abstract

Age-related immune dysfunction has been confirmed by many studies. All of these changes result in increased susceptibility to infectious diseases and pathological conditions associated with inflammation or autoreactivity. To prevent these changes, we used various model approaches as follows: (i) the models of hematopoietic stem cells (HSCs) transplantation in irradiated chimeras, (ii) the model of heterochronic parabiosis that provides regular physiological exchange by blood factors between partners, and (iii) cocultivation of lymphoid cells and niche-forming cells in vitro to determine its intercellular communication mechanisms. It was shown that the old HSCs equally effectively restore the immune system of young animals and their own. But, the young hematopoietic cells behaved like old in the old organism. Parabiosis model demonstrated that regular exchange by blood factors between heterochronic partners does not lead to the old system rejuvenation. And we observed impaired capacity of splenic $CD11c^{+}$ DC and macrophages from young heterochronic parabionts to co-stimulate proliferation of T-cells in vitro with statistically significant decrease in nuclear factor-kappa B (NFκB) p65 and increased expression of IκBα during early activation events. These findings suggest that age-related changes in the immune system are multifactor process, and whole-system environment of the organism plays a crucial role in the occurrence of age-related immune system alterations.

Keywords: immune system, T-cell, heterochronic chimeras, aging, parabiosis

1. Introduction

The immune system is a powerful barrier that protects the organism from the damaging factors of various origins: microorganisms, viruses, transformed cells, and tissues. Tumors, as well as damaged and aged cells, are damaging factors that appear throughout the life. It is known that the incidence of various infectious diseases, autoimmune diseases, and cancer increases with age. It is expected that these changes can be caused by age-related disorders of the immune system. The relationship between the occurrence of age-related diseases with defects in the immune system has led to the hypothesis that the aging of the immune system can trigger development of most age-related diseases. For this reason, great emphasis is paid to study aging processes of the immune system.

The aging of the immune system is the most striking example of the changes that occur in the aging. Age-related changes in the immune system begin to develop very early, still in puberty [1, 2]. Age-related disorders are observed in the functioning of many types of lymphoid cells, but the most significant changes occur in the population of T-lymphocytes. It is known that the T-cell response in the elderly is accompanied by breach of lymphocyte's ability to transmit intracellular signals, reduction in diversity repertoire of T-cell receptor, decrease the proliferative response on antigen stimulation (response to antigens, mitogens, lectins, antibodies to CD3, etc.), and changes in the repertoire of produced cytokines [1].

The study of age-related changes in the immune system certainly gives rise to the question: due to what parts of the immune system are experiencing these violations? It is known that immune function is carried out by cells that are continuously updated in the body, passing through the stages of hematopoietic stem cells of bone marrow (BM) to highly differentiated immunocompetent cells: different subpopulations of T-lymphocytes, B-lymphocytes, and monocyte-macrophages. The lifespan of most of these cells depending upon the type and a functional feature ranges from several days to several months or even years. But, the duration of life is relatively short when compared with the duration of life of the organism in which they function [3].

Investigation of age-related disorders in the function of hematopoietic stem cells has shown that with aging the amount of B-lymphocyte progenitor cells reduces [4], such as diversity of B-cell repertoire in the mouse bone marrow [5]. For T-cell, the main factor that contributes to the reduction in T-lymphopoiesis with age is the thymic atrophy [1]. At the same time, more recent studies have shown that reducing the production of naïve lymphocytes with age is also dependent on intracellular changes in hematopoietic stem cells. It is known that old HSCs after transplantation to the young lethally irradiated mice can restore hematopoiesis with "aged" properties, including a reduced ability to generate T-cells [4, 6]. Reducing the number of B- and T-lymphocyte progenitor cells changes the cellular composition of hematopoietic system, which leads to the relative dominance of myeloid cells, often called age-dependent myeloid skewed or offset [4, 6, 7].

It is assumed that trigger of the immune system dysfunction is age-related involution of the thymus. T-progenitor cells that migrated to the thymus from the bone marrow pass difficult way of "training" with a tight positive and negative selection. Only a small proportion of T-lymphocytes differentiates and migrates from the thymus to peripheral lymphoid organs. With aging, there is a loss of thymic epithelium, and as a result, defects occur in the maturation and differentiation of progenitors of T-lymphocytes. Additionally, the thymus is a target for various pathogens that utilize it for their persistence and affect editing repertoire of naïve T-cells [8].

With aging, there are several types of changes in the functioning of T-cells including the decrease in the proliferative response after T-cell receptor (TCR)/cluster of differentiation 3 (CD3) activation, expansion memory cells, and simultaneous reduction in the number of naïve T-cells and the accumulation of CD28-T-cells. Though the mechanism of age changes is not fully known, the change in intracellular signaling associated with the TCR/CD3 complex is regarded as the most significant damaging factor [9].

Key sources of the above factors, which regulate the functioning of T-cells, are elements of their microenvironment (niche) in the lymphoid organs. Microenvironmental cells include fibroblasts and antigen-presenting cells (APCs hereinafter), particularly macrophages and dendritic cells (DCs hereinafter), which play a key role in the proliferation and function of T-lymphocytes. It is known that the ability of dendritic cells to stimulate an immune response to the antigens decreases with age. It also reduces the ability of dendritic cells and macrophages to stimulate protective anti-tumor immune response. But information about age-related changes in the co-stimulatory properties of lymphoid niche cells is now somewhat contradictory as a whole [10, 11].

Thus, the mechanism of changes in the functions of the immune system in aging involves three main components that affect the function: age of hematopoietic stem progenitor cells, age of lymphoid organs microenvironment, and the impact of the overall environment of the old organism on the development of immune responses.

To isolate the effects of these components and to establish mechanisms of age dysfunction of the immune system, we use artificial models of biological systems, composed of elements of different ages, the so-called heterochronic chimeras. We used three main approaches to the study of the mechanisms of age-related changes in the immune system: (1) study of the role of the aging of hematopoietic stem cell disorders in the immune system on the model of lethally irradiated heterochronic chimeras; (2) study of the role of the system environment on the model heterochronic parabiosis, which provides a full exchange with growth, hormonal factors, and blood cells between animals of different ages; and (3) study of disorders of the lymphoid cell niche in reducing immune function with aging.

2. The aging of the immune system and approaches to its rejuvenation

2.1. Investigation of the effect of hematopoietic stem cells aging on the immune system functions in lethally irradiated heterochronic chimeras

Animals that underwent lethal irradiation generally show 100% destruction of lymphoid and hematopoietic stem cells in the organism and the complete immune dysfunction causes the death within 10–14 days. Replacement of dead cells on donor hematopoietic stem cells results in the restoration of HSCs pool in the bone marrow and immune system functions. All lymphoid cells in thus chimeras are of donor origin.

Thus, we used this model to identify the age differences of the regenerative properties of HSCs, and to elucidate the ability of stem cells to restore the immune system of old animals.

Parameters	Experimental groups					
	Y (n = 8)	Yy (n = 10)	Yo (n = 14)	O (n = 7)	Oy (n = 10)	Oo (n = 7)
Thymus mass, mg	34.6 ± 2.1	18.1* ± 2.4	17.7* ± 3.8	12.5* ± 1.3	6.4**,# ± 0.3	8.2***,#,## ± 0.5
Thy 1.2⁺splenocytes, %	56.3 ± 2.3	49.4* ± 1.9	42.3*,** ± 2.1	35.2* ± 1.3	28.3**,# ± 3.2	37.3## ± 2.6
CD4⁺ splenocytes, %	39.3 ± 2.2	38.3 ± 2.3	32.8* ± 1.9	23.4* ± 1.2	22.7** ± 2.3	25.9 ± 2.6
CD8⁺ splenocytes, %	17.3 ± 1.4	13.3 ± 0.6	11.2*,** ± 0.5	15.1 ± 1.0	7.7**,# ± 0.5	15.3**,## ± 0.4
CD4⁺ CD44⁺ splenocytes, %[1]	27.5 ± 2.0	27.4 ± 0.7	33.0** ± 2.5	69.7* ± 5.2	61.2*,** ± 3.7	58.7*,*** ± 5.4
IgM⁺ splenocytes, %	37.8 ± 2.2	39.7 ± 2.0	47.5 ± 2.4	59.3* ± 3.6	57.6** ± 3.1	55.1 ± 2.4

Table 1. Thymus weight and number of lymphocyte subpopulations in the spleen of mice different experimental groups, M ± SE.

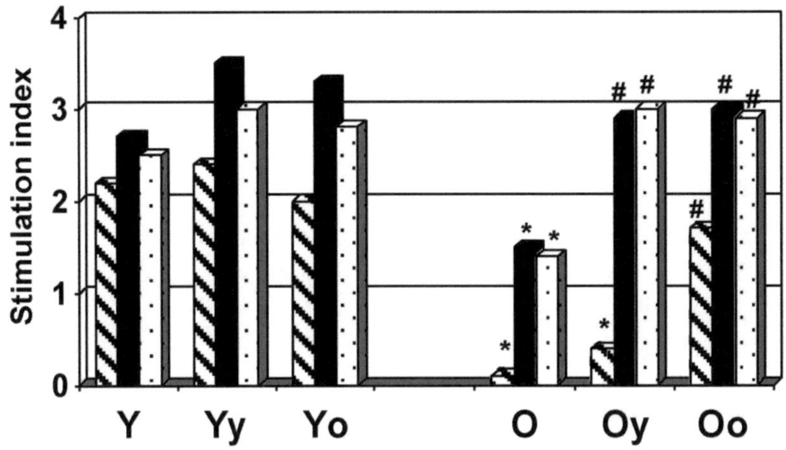

Figure 1. Proliferative response of splenocytes after mitogen stimulation in vitro.The shaded bars, PHA response (10 μg/ml); dark bars, Con A response (5 μg/ml); the spotted bars, LPS response (30 μg/ml). Symbol of the experimental groups: Y, young intact mice; Yy, young irradiated animals which were recovered of BM cells from young mice; Yo, young irradiated animals which were recovered of BM cells from old mice; O, old intact mice; Oy, old irradiated animals which were recovered of BM cells from young mice; Oo, old irradiated animals which were recovered of BM cells from old mice. CBA/Ca female mice were irradiated and recovered of 15 × 10^6 BM cells at 4 (young) and 22 (old) months of age. At 3 months after the recovering mice were euthanized and immune parameters were analyzed. *, P (t) < 0.05 comparing young intact animals; #, P (t) < 0.05 comparing old intact animals. The mice number in each group is at least 8.

Studies were conducted on female CBA/Ca mice, where the age of the recipients and donors was 4 months (young) and 22 months (old) before the start of the experiment. For 3 h prior to administration of HSCs, mice of recipients were irradiated with X-ray radiation dose of 8.5 Gy (dose rate of 0.72 Gy/min). To eliminate mature T-lymphocytes, donor bone marrow cells were treated with monoclonal antibodies to the Thy1.2 mouse antigen. Bone marrow cells were

http://dx.doi.org/10.5772/64046

administered intravenously at a dose of 15 × 10^6 per mouse. Immunological parameters were tested for 3 months after irradiation and bone marrow transplantation.

Mice were divided into six groups: (1) young intact animals (Y), (2) young irradiated animals that were administered BM cells from young mice (Yy), (3) young irradiated animals that were administered BM cells from old mice (Yo), (4) old intact animals (O), (5) irradiated old animals that were administered BM cells from young mice (Oy), and (6) old irradiated animals that were administered BM cells from old mice (Oo). Functional status of the immune system was evaluated by the following parameters: the weight of the thymus, the number of leukocytes in the blood, the number of lymphocyte subpopulations in the spleen using flow cytometry and antibodies to the mouse antigens CD4, CD8, IgM, CD44 (Sigma, USA), and the proliferative activity of splenocytes in vitro in response to mitogens phytohemagglutinin (PHA), concanavalin A (Con A), and lipopolysaccharide (LPS).

It is known that the immune system of old animals is different from the young in many investigated indices. Particularly, thymus weight and the number of white blood cells are significantly reduced in old individuals. Moreover, the number of $CD4^+$ cells and the $CD4^+/CD8^+$ ratio in the spleen are decreased in aged animals. Lymphocytes with a phenotype of memory T-cells (CD4 $^+$CD44$^+$) increases in old animals are approximately twice higher. These changes in subpopulations of T-cells significantly affect their functional properties. For instance, lymphocytes of old animals respond poorly to T-lymphocyte antigens PHA response and Con A response. Response to LPS response (B-lymphocyte-specific mitogen) also significantly reduced with age, despite the high content of B-cells in the spleens of old mice CBA/Ca. Other authors [1, 5] also observed similar changes in the composition and functions of the spleen cells of old mice. We performed the experiments of heterochronic transplantation of BM cells with irradiated CBA/Ca mice. The results are shown in **Table 1** and **Figure 1**. We can find out the following interesting changes.

First, the changes were caused by transplantation procedure itself. Significant reduction in thymus weight to all exposed mice was observed possibly as a result of the effect of prolonged stress and radiation damage (**Table 1**). In young recipients, the number of T-cells in the spleen was also decreased (**Table 1**). Otherwise, in old recipients, transplantation of BM cells (irrespective of donor age) led to an increase in the proliferative response to mitogens. For example, the splenocyte response to Con A and LPS in old recipients reached the level of young mouse (**Figure 1**).

The second type of changes has occurred in an organism the young recipients after injection the old BM cells (Yo group). In particular, we observed a decrease in the content of Thy 1.2+ lymphocytes perhaps by increasing the number of CD8+ cells in the spleen (**Table 1**). Yo group showed an increased content of IgM+ cells and increased number of CD4+CD44+ memory-like cells in the spleen (**Table 1**). These data are confirmed by many other studies, which reveal HSCs dysfunctions with age [7, 8].

CBA/Ca female mice were irradiated and recovered of 15 × 10^6 BM cells at 4 (young) and 22 (old) months of age. After 3 months, the recovering mice were euthanized and subjected to immune parameter analysis. Symbol of the experimental groups: Y, young intact mice; Yy, young irradiated animals that were recovered of BM cells from young mice; Yo, young irradiated animals that were recovered of BM cells from old mice; O, old intact mice; Oy, old irradiated animals that were recovered of BM cells from young mice; and Oo, old irradiated animals that were recovered of BM cells from old mice.

*, $P(t) < 0.05$ comparing young intact animals.

**, $P(t) < 0.05$ comparing young irradiated animals recovered of young BM cells.

***, $P(t) < 0.05$ comparing young irradiated animals recovered of old BM cells.

#, $P(t) < 0.05$ comparing old intact animals.

##, $P(t) < 0.05$ comparing old irradiated animals recovered of young BM cells.

###, $P(t) < 0.05$ comparing old irradiated animals recovered of old BM cells.

It should be noted that we did not detect the rejuvenation effect of a young bone marrow cells on the old immune system functions. The third change is caused by the systemic factors of organism. Major parameters—thymus mass, number of T-cells in the spleen, contents of $CD4^+$ lymphocytes, response to T-cell mitogens, number of IgM+, and $CD4^+CD44^+$ lymphocytes —in young recipients remained as high as those in young intact individual. Mice of Oy group showed lower weight of the thymus and decreased number of CD8+ cells in the spleen compared to animal group Oo (**Table 1** and **Figure 1**). The obtained data may suggest that young hematopoietic cells may decrease the ability for their comprehensive development in old recipients compared to their own old hematopoietic cells (**Table 1** and **Figure 1**). Furthermore, an increased level of $CD4^+CD44^+$ splenocytes in Oy mice is an interesting fact. It is known that the number of T-cells with memory phenotype steadily increases with age. It is supposed that the differentiation of naïve T-lymphocytes in memory T-cells can be induced by repeating antigenic load as well as a chronic inflammation (inflammaging) in the old body [9]. Therefore, high level of memory-like cells in old recipient may suggest that the macroenvironment of old organism can specifically stimulate the differentiation and accumulation of cells with memory phenotype, regardless of the "age" of hematopoietic stem cells.

The results of this study not only confirmed the known information about the changes of the immune system with aging but also gave new information about the possible mechanisms of age-related dysfunction. It should be noted that the residence of young cells/tissues in an old body leads to a deterioration of their functional properties in most studies using heterochronic chimeras [12–15].

In our study of young hematopoietic cells were also unable to improve any of the investigated parameters of the immune system in old animals. Thus, we examined the number of antibody-forming cells to sheep red blood cells (SRBCs). The immune response to thymus-dependent antigens is not affected by the age of HSCs, but depended on the age of the recipients (**Figure 2**). In young recipients, on the contrary, the immune response of Yy and Yo showed similar strength to that of young intact mice (Y). This fact may suggest that the age-related change of HSCs functions is not a key factor in the occurrence of age-related dysfunction of the immune system.

http://dx.doi.org/10.5772/64046

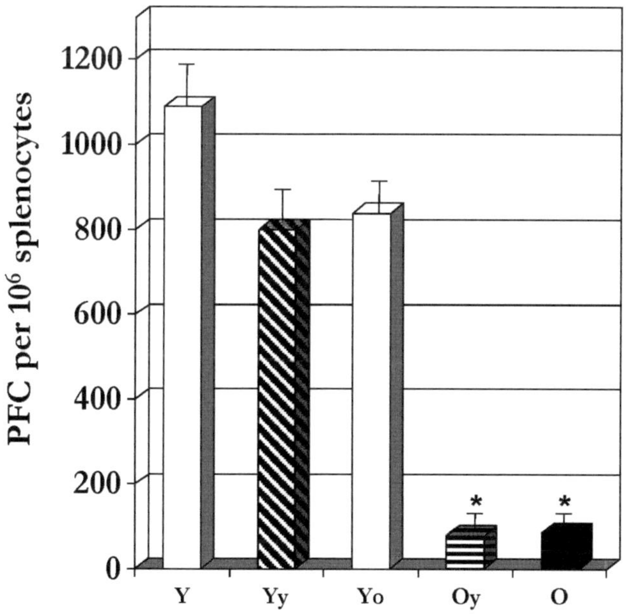

Figure 2. The number of antibody-forming cells to SRBCs in the spleen of immunized CBA/Ca experimental mice.Symbol of the experimental groups: Y, young intact mice; Yy, young irradiated animals which were recovered of BM cells from young mice; Yo, young irradiated animals which were recovered of BM cells from old mice; O, old intact mice; Oy, old irradiated animals which were recovered of BM cells from young mice. CBA/Ca female mice were irradiated and recovered of 15 × 10^6 BM cells at 3 (young) and 24 (old) months of age. At 3 months after the recovering mice were immunized of 10^8 SRBCs intraperitonealy. Four days after animals were euthanized and subjected to immune parameter analysis. *, P (t) < 0.05 comparing young intact animals; #, P (t) < 0.05 comparing old intact animals. The mice number in each group is at least 8.

Consequently, we could identify the following age-related differences in the regenerative properties of HSCs. HSCs of old mice have a reduced ability to produce Thy 1.2$^+$ cells, CD4$^+$, and CD8$^+$ cells but fully recovered the ability to develop an immune response to SRBCs in young recipients. Transplantation of HSCs of old mice results in the opposite effect in old individuals: it led to accumulation of more Thy 1.2$^+$ and CD8$^+$ cells, and more significant proliferative response of splenocytes to PHA was observed (**Figure 1** and **Table 1**). However, these changes do not result in the restoration of immune response to SRBCs. These results may suggest that the differentiation of HSCs is affected by some factors present in the microenvironment of lymphoid organs, where HSCs are maturated. To elucidate this hypothesis, we used another model—heterochronic parabiosis—which is described in the next chapter.

2.2. Study of the mechanisms of age-related changes in the immune system on the model heterochronic parabiosis

The parabiosis model represents a pair of animals in which the common blood circulation is established by a surgical procedure. In fact, this model allows creating Siamese twins surgically in experimental conditions [16]. The model of parabiosis is actively studied in recent years. It was shown that the mutual exchange of progenitor cells of fibroblast/myofibroblasts [17, 18], hematopoietic [19, 20] and non-hematopoietic stem cells [21], and the endothelial progenitor cells [22] actively occurs between partners due to the general bloodstream.

We evaluated the status of the immune system in heterochronic parabionts 3 months after the operation [23]. We assumed that the migration of young stem cells in combination with young serum factors will contribute to restoration of the structure and function of the thymus in old animals. The rejuvenation of the thymus, in turn, will lead to restoration of function and the repertoire of T-cells in peripheral lymphoid organs and the rejuvenation of the immune system of old parabiotic partners.

Disturbances of thymic function with age are well known. It is found that the age-induced thymus atrophy is accompanied by a reduction in thymocyte number and a decrease in T-cell progenitors in the bone marrow. These disturbances can be induced by changes in the hormonal balance, for example, increased levels of sex steroids with age [24]. When using the model heterochronic parabiosis, we suggested that the young blood will improve the function of the thymus in the old animals. As a result, we have not found improved indices in thymus parameters of old partners. Furthermore, we obtained a decrease in thymus weight in young heterochronic partner without significant changes in thymocyte subpopulation number [23].

To assess changes in the T-cell functions, we evaluated the parameters that are most significantly changed during aging: CD4 and CD8 T-cell subpopulations in the spleen, and the proliferative activity of splenocytes in response to mitogens in vitro [25]. It was shown that the proliferative activity of splenocytes in response to PHA in vitro was not restored in old heterochronic partners, and decreased in the young ones after 3 months of coexistence. Similar changes have been identified in the $CD4^+$ and $CD8^+$ T-cell subpopulation numbers in the spleen. The CD4/CD8 ratio did not change the spleen of old partners and significantly decreased in the young ones. Furthermore, it has been shown that the amount of the cells with memory phenotype ($CD44^+$) was increased in young partners to the level of old animals (**Table 2**).

Parameters	**Experimental groups**			
	Young isochronic (n = 8)	**Young heterochronic (n = 8)**	**Old heterochronic (n = 8)**	**Old isochronic (n = 10)**
Splenocytes number, 10^6	153.60 ± 16.56	150.00 ± 11.21	118.80 ± 9.60	90.80 ± 12.53^a
Bone marrow cell number, 10^6 per femur	17.38 ± 1.05	14.88 ± 1.39	14.81 ± 2.26	17.81 ± 1.06
Proliferative activity in vitro, stimulation index	1.71 ± 0.15	1.32 ± 0.13*	1.59 ± 0.25	1.39 ± 0.07^a
Phagocytic macrophages, %	63.00 ± 2.57	50.00 ± 3.32**	48.38 ± 3.75	52.40 ± 2.17^{aa}
$CD4^+$ cell number in the spleen, %	22.10 ± 0.91	19.16 ± 1.93	22.54 ± 2.36	20.63 ± 2.16
$CD8^+$ cell number in the spleen, %	9.75 ± 0.91	16.23 ± 1.75**	15.34 ± 0.54	12.70 ± 1.22

Parameters	Experimental groups			
	Young isochronic (n = 8)	Young heterochronic (n = 8)	Old heterochronic (n = 8)	Old isochronic (n = 10)
CD4/CD8 ratio in the spleen	2.51 ± 0.42	1.27 ± 0.20*	1.49 ± 0.18	1.62 ± 0.05[aa]
$CD4^+44^+$ cell number in the spleen, %	14.32 ± 1.34	21.58 ± 0.34**	23.86 ± 1.29	18.74 ± 1.38[a]
$CD8^+44^+$ cell number in the spleen, %	0.96 ± 0.23	2.21 ± 0.66*	2.42 ± 0.40	1.87 ± 0.25[a]
$CD4^+25^+$ cell number in the spleen, %	2.41 ± 0.25	1.81 ± 0.38	1.93 ± 0.47	3.25 ± 1.25
$CD4^+25^+FoxP3^+$ cell number in the spleen, %	0.17 ± 0.06	0.09 ± 0.04	0.06 ± 0.03*	0.48 ± 0.25

Table 2. Effects of heterochronic parabiosis on the immunological parameters of CBA/Ca mice, M ± SE.

For the parabiosis, CBA/Ca male mice were typically joined at 2–3 (young) and 22–23 (old) months of age. At 3 months after the parabiosis initiation, mice were euthanized and subjected to immune parameter analysis. All pairs with tumors were excluded from the study. *, $p(t) < 0.05$ comparing isochronic animals of the same age; **, $p(t) < 0.01$ comparing isochronic animals of the same age, a, $p(t) < 0.05$ comparing young isochronic animals; aa, $p(t) < 0.01$ comparing young isochronic animals.

The most optimistic result in such a pessimistic picture was shown by regulatory T-cells—their number decreased significantly in the old heterochronic partners to young level (**Table 2**).

Thus, at this stage of study it was found that the mutual exchange of blood between heterochronic partners did not result in recovery of the thymus, the peripheral T-cell number, and immune functions normalizing in aged parabiotic partners. Major changes have been observed in young partners. There was a decrease of thymus weight, disorders of peripheral T-cell repertoire, and a decrease in PHA-stimulated lymphocyte proliferation in vitro. In fact, we observed age-related changes in the immune system of young heterochronic partners in accelerated rate.

This model of accelerated aging of the immune system has provided us with a unique opportunity to trace the dynamics of the appearance of age-related changes in the immune system. We examined the changes in immune functions in young heterochronic partners at different time points—3, 6, and 12 weeks after surgery. We found that the first change, which occurs in young heterochronic partners, was doubling number of $CD8^+44^+$cells in the spleen 3 weeks after surgery. After 6 weeks, the rate of this index remained at a high level, and there was also a significant decrease in CD4/CD8 ratio in the spleen. At the 12th week of coexistence, a decrease in the proliferative response of T-cells in response to PHA, as well as significantly decreased number of phagocytic cells in the spleen, was found [23].

Increasing the number of $CD8^+44^+$ memory-like cells in the spleen is the first change of a young partner. The study of lymphoid cell migration between the heterochronic partners has shown that an increasing number of $CD8^{+}44^{+}$ cells may be mediated by an increase in the number of young $CD8^{+}44^{+}$ cells in the spleen, bone marrow, and thymus of old partners [23]. We hypothesized that these changes may have multiple mechanisms of occurrence: the migration of young $CD8^{+}44^{+}$ cells to the old partner, or the proliferation of young cells into the old body through antigen-specific or homeostatic proliferation. However, we cannot assert which of the proposed mechanisms is the key in age-related changes on the basis of the obtained results.

The population of $CD8^{+}44^{+}$ memory-like cells is short-lived and quickly proliferating. It is assumed that a shorter time $CD8^{+}44^{+}$ T-cell recycling relative to naïve $CD8^{+}$ T-cells is associated with the higher speed of their homeostatic proliferation [26]. At the same time, in aged mice, the reduction in the turnover of memory-like $CD44^{+}CD8+$ cells was found. The authors suggested that the reduced turnover of aged $CD44^{+}$ $CD8^{+}$ cells reflected an inhibitory influence of the aged environment, including APCs [27–29]. The presented data may indicate that the old lymphoid microenvironment can induce changes in the differentiation and functioning of $CD8^{+}$ T-cells. We suggested that the rapid growth of the number of $CD8^{+}44^{+}$ cells in young heterochronic partners may result from the mutual influence of the two environments—young for fast proliferation and old for $CD8^{+}44^{+}$ memory cell differentiation.

The obtained data indicate that our hypothesis—that the mechanisms of the immune aging can be mediated by dysfunctions of lymphoid cells and organs (thymus, bone marrow) or insufficient production of some factors (hormones, cytokines, and growth factors)—is unfounded. The obtained results showed that the general circulation between partners of different ages, which provides a mutual exchange of hematopoietic stem cells, naïve lymphocytes, hormones, cytokines, and growth factors, does not lead to the restoration of the old immune system functioning. On the contrary, it was found that the common bloodstream from the old to the young partner is able to induce the aging of a young immune system. It is assumed that changes in the proliferation and differentiation of young $CD8^{+}$ T-cells, which presumably enhanced by their homeostatic proliferation, appear due to the influence of the old lymphoid niches. To test this hypothesis, we used the model of heterochronic cocultivation of lymphocytes with cells that form spleen lymphoid niche (macrophages or CD $11c^{+}$ dendritic cells).

2.3. The study of age-related changes of lymphoid niche cells in the model of heterochronic parabiosis

It is well known that peripheral T-cell functions are regulated by multiple extrinsic factors, in particular by the microenvironment of lymphoid organs, where T-cells usually form special zones such as a periarteriolar lymphoid sheath in the spleen. T-cell activities in these zones are regulated by cells of their niche. Lymphoid niche includes fibroblastic reticular cells, which organize T-cell zones and antigen-presenting cells. APCs are important T-cell regulators and include a broad variety of different cell types such as dendritic cells, B-cells, and macrophages. Dendritic cells are professional APCs and regulatory cells, and are able to either induce tolerance or stimulate profound immune response in an organism [30]. Macrophages can also display some DC-like features [31]. APCs are composed of a very heterogeneous population of cells and they all can significantly affect T-cell functions. APCs can regulate T-cell functions through multiple mechanisms, particularly through the action of paracrine factors (cytokines) and through co-stimulatory or inhibitory surface molecules.

The study of DC and macrophage functions is a very difficult task, since in situ these cells are part of an extremely complex structure, forming lymphoid organ stromal microenvironment. It makes it almost impossible to evaluate their native functions in vivo. Therefore, we have created in vitro system to assess the co-stimulatory properties of individual types of lymphoid stromal cells. For investigation, we chose macrophages and DC of the spleen, which are able to influence the antigen-specific and homeostatic proliferation of T-cells. To assess its functions, we have chosen the model of coculturing APCs with purified T-cells in vitro after stimulation by PHA. To determine the overall effect of heterochronic parabiosis on APCs, we evaluated PHA-mediated T-cell stimulation in the presence of a particular type of APCs—either total population of CD11c$^+$ splenic dendritic cells or enriched macrophage population (splenic adherent cells).

T-cells are stimulated via binding of PHA (T-cell superantigen) with T-cell receptor, which results in polyclonal activation of T-cells. The procedure is simple and reliable to determine T-cell antigen-induced proliferation because it mimics the binding of presented antigen with T-cell receptor [32] which does not involve direct artificial activation of intracellular signal cascades.

T-cells were isolated from the total suspension of splenocytes using columns with nylon wool (Polyscience, Inc.) according to the manufacturer's instruction. Flow cytometry analysis of enriched T-cell suspension (stained by anti-CD3-FITC monoclonal antibody (Pickcell Laboratory, the Netherlands) indicated 90–95% purity. Dendritic cells were isolated from the spleen by a CD11c$^+$ selection magnetic separation kit EasySep (Stemcell Technology) according to the manufacturer's instruction. The total population of enriched splenic macrophages was harvested from the splenocytes by adhesion to plastic according to the routine method [23].

Coculturing experiments were carried out to examine the capability of total splenic macrophages and dendritic cells to co-stimulate T-cell proliferation. Coculture experiments included the following combinations: (1) purified splenic T-cells from control young intact mice were cocultured with enriched population of splenic dendritic cells of parabionts, (2) purified splenic T-cells from control young intact mice were cocultured with enriched population of splenic macrophages of parabionts, (3) purified splenic T-cells from parabionts were cocultured with enriched population of autologous splenic dendritic cells, and (4) purified splenic T-cells from parabionts were cocultured with enriched population of autologous splenic macrophages.

The results of experiment are shown in **Figure 3**. First, we tested PHA-mediated proliferative response of native splenocytes or purified T-cells alone to check the background values, and observed significant differences between young and old isochronic parabionts (**Figure 3A** and **B**, $P(t) < 0.05$). The splenocyte proliferation rate in young and old heterochronic parabionts (Yo and Oy) did not differ from the rates of young or old isochronic controls (Yy and Oo). Otherwise, we observed a decrease in proliferative capacity of purified splenic T-cells in the heterochronic parabionts (Yo and Oy) compared to young isochronic control (Yy) (**Figure 3B**, $P(t) < 0.05$).

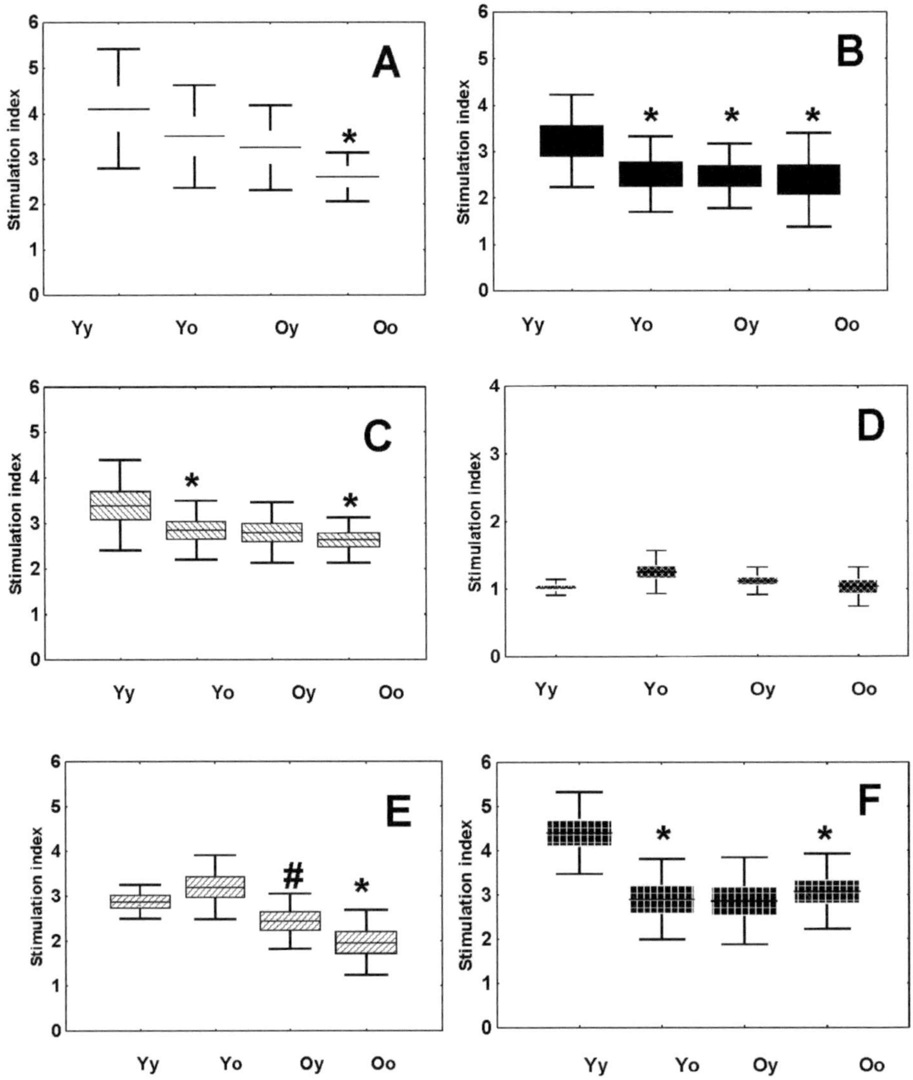

Figure 3. Proliferative response of purified splenic T-cells after PHA stimulation in vitro.Symbol of the experimental groups: Yy, young isochronic animals; Yo, young heretochronic animals; Oy, old heterochronic mice; Oo, old isochronic mice. CBA/Ca female mice at 1.5 months after the parabiosis initiation was euthanized and subjected to analysis. All pairs with tumors were excluded from the study. **A.** Proliferative activity of native splenocytes. **B.** Proliferative activity of purified splenic T-cells. **C.** Proliferative activity of purified young control T-cells cocultivated with $CD11c^{+}$ DC from mice of different experimental groups. **D.** Proliferative activity of purified young control T-cells cocultivated with adherent splenic cells from mice of different experimental groups. **E.** Proliferative activity of purified splenic T-cells cocultivated with autologous $CD11c^{+}$ DC from experimental mice. **F.** Proliferative activity of purified splenic T-cells cocultivated with autologous adherent splenic cells from experimental mice. *, $P(t) < 0.05$ comparing young isochronic animals; #, $P(t) < 0.05$ comparing old intact animals. The mice number in each group is at least 8.

http://dx.doi.org/10.5772/64046

Although the interaction of T-cells usually involves great number of soluble and surface co-stimulatory molecules, we examined the effect of cocultivation of splenic DCs and macrophages on PHA-induced T-cell activation.

We used two approaches to assess the activity of spleen dendritic cells and macrophages. The first approach is to assess the age-related APC changes in spleen microenvironment, so we studied the effect of DC and macrophages on the proliferation of intact young T-cells. As shown in **Figure 3C**, we observed significant decrease in the proliferative capacity of enriched population of young intact T-cells, which were cocultivated with CD11c$^+$ DCs of young heterochronic parabionts, but the value was almost same as the cells cocultured with old ones (**Figure 3C**, $P(U) < 0.05$). Therefore, we observed the impairment of CD11c$^+$ DC functions for maintaining the proliferation of young T-cells in the group of young heterochronic parabionts. When macrophages were cocultured, we found no similar changes (**Figure 3D**).

Second, we investigated the activation of T-cells by cocultivation with their own dendritic cells or macrophages (autologous mouse) to determine which APC have an inhibitory effect on the activation of T-cells in heterochronic parabionts. As shown in **Figure 3E**, a significant decrease in the proliferation rate of T-cells from old isochronic parabionts cocultured with autologous DCs was observed as compared to the young isochronic ones. Meanwhile, no decrease was observed in the proliferation rate of T-cells cocultured with total splenic dendritic cells from young heterochronic parabionts to the level of young isochronic parabionts. We also analyzed the influence of the total population of splenic adherent cells from animals of different experimental groups on the T-cell proliferation in vitro (**Figure 3F**). The proliferative capacity of T-cells from young heterochronic partners, which were cocultured with their own splenic adherent cells, was found to drop to the level of old animals as compared to young isochronic partners ($P(t) < 0.05$). Thus, we suggest that the T-cell proliferative capacity can be strongly impacted by niche-forming cells and their age-related changes can cause T-cell dysfunction. Macrophages could act as T-cell dysfunction inducers in our experimental model of heterochronic parabiosis.

Finally, we examined key mechanisms of T-cell activation. It has been investigated as complicated mechanism which includes both the activation process and the apoptosis of activated lymphocytes [32]. We examined the expression of RelA , IkBα, and caspase p20 during the activation of T-cells.

Figure 4 shows the RelA, IkBα, and caspase p20 expression of splenic T-cells. The amount of those proteins was determined by using Western blotting method. Coculture with macrophage was used for the experiments because most significant differences were observed. By 2 h of cocultivation of T-cell with macrophages from spleens of autologous donors, a decreased level of RelA and caspase 3 p20 protein in old isochronic parabionts versus the young ones was observed (**Figure 4A** and **C**, respectively, $P(U) < 0.05$). In young heterochronic parabionts, T-cell cocultivation with macrophages led to another effect—the RelA level also reduced whereas caspase 3, p20 protein remained unchanged in this group (**Figure 4A** and **C**, respectively, $P(U) < 0.05$). However, neither significant changes in the IκBα level (**Figure 4B**) nor any sign of expression of the full (not active) form of caspase 3 in T-cells was detected (data not presented).

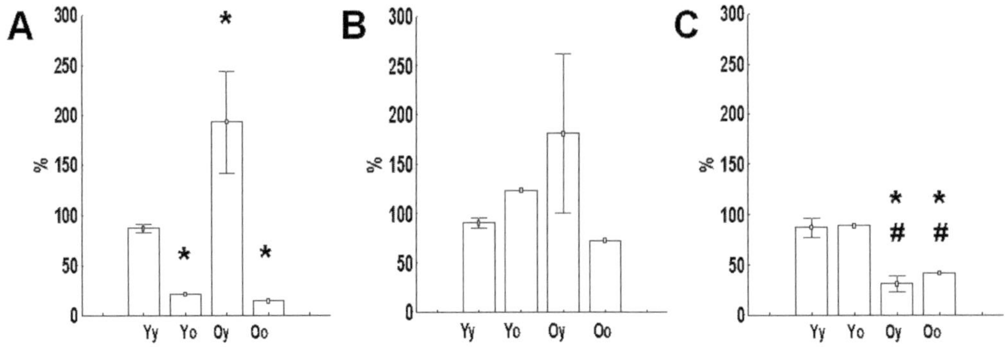

Figure 4. Level of RelA, IkBα, and caspase p20 in purified splenic T-cells from parabiotic mice after 2 h of coculturing with splenic macrophage-rich population of adherent cells from animals of the same experimental groups.The total splenic T-cells from parabionts were isolated and 10×10^6 cells were cocultured with previously enriched total splenic macrophages from 10×10^7 splenocytes of mice of the same experimental groups. PHA of 10 μg/ml was added to cell suspensions, and they had been stimulated for 2 h. Then, cells were lysed, and the total cellular extract had been analyzed with Western blotting for the main components of T-cell activation signalling: RelA (A), IkBα (B), caspase p20 (C). Data are presented from results of at least three experiments. *, $P(U) < 0.05$ compared to young isochronic parabionts; #, $P(U) < 0.05$ compared to young heterochronic parabionts.

Moreover, the experiment of 18 h of cocultivation was performed. By 18 h, we observed equalization of the RelA protein level between T-cells from all experimental groups. No considerable changes in the expression level of the IκBα protein in activated T-cells from different experimental groups were marked in this stage of activation. However, the level of the activated form of caspase 3 (p20) was still considerably higher in T-cells from young isochronic and young heterochronic parabionts in comparison with T-cells from either old isochronic or heterochronic parabiotic animals [33].

The experiment focused merely on the key factors of T-cell activation during APC co-stimulation, and we found out considerable changes in the expression level of several key proteins for T-cell mitogen-induced proliferation. We notice that splenic macrophages can impact T-cell proliferation and mitogen-activated T-cell signaling.

3. Conclusions

Adaptive immune response most markedly declines with age and main reasons for that are atrophy of the thymus that begins immediately after puberty, and massive changes in the T-cell compartment of lymphoid organs [2]. Defects in T-cell functions greatly affect protective capabilities of an organism so that it becomes more susceptible to different pathogens and cancer [1, 34].

Numerous attempts to rejuvenate the immune system have shown that processes of age-related changes in T-cell functions are rather complex. Moreover, an interchange between the young immune system and the old one established via the common blood cell circulation induced an age-related decline in the young immune parameters [13].

In the present study, we examined the mechanisms of age-related dysfunction of the immune system using various models of heterochronic chimeras, and analyzing the interaction of various parts of the immune system: hematopoietic stem cells, lymphoid organ microenvironment, lymphocytes, and systemic factors that circulate in the blood.

Using model of the irradiated chimera, we found that the old hematopoietic stem cells after 3 months residing in lethally irradiated young organism lead to the formation of a smaller amount of $CD4^+$ and $CD8^+$ T-cells in the spleen of young animals than of young HSCs. These data are confirmed by many other studies that reveal a violation of HSCs functioning with age [4, 5]. But the purpose of our study was not to study individual changes of HSCs functions, but the contribution of these changes to the age-related dysfunction of the immune system. According to our findings, changes in the functional properties of old HSCs do not exercise a significant influence on the amplitude of humoral immune response in young animals (**Figure 2**, Yo group). This fact may suggest that the age-related changes in the HSCs cannot cause age-related disorders of the immune system. This supposition is also confirmed by the results, which show that old HSCs lead to a more significant proliferative response of splenocytes to PHA in old animals when compared with young HSCs (**Figure 1**).

Next, we used another model—heterochronic parabiosis. This model is characterized by a common blood circulation between animals of different ages, allowing them to share not only stem cells but also blood lymphocytes and circulated growth factors and hormones. But instead of the regeneration of the immune system in old partner, we observed the progressive reduction of the most immunological parameters in young ones in this model.

Accelerated aging of the immune system in young heterochronic partners gave us a unique opportunity in a short time to study the trigger mechanism of these age-related changes. It was determined that the first change appeared within 3 weeks after surgery is the doubled number of $CD8^+44^+$ memory-like cells in the spleen of young heterochronic partners that reached a level in old mice. Increasing the number of these cells may indicate that there is one possible mechanism of age-related dysfunction of the immune system in heterochronic parabiosis. Since the differentiation of $CD8^+44^+$ T-cells is provided by their homeostatic proliferation in the peripheral lymphoid organs, we assume that these changes can occur as a result of enhancing their homeostatic proliferation under the influence of old lymphoid niches.

It has been well known that the functioning of T-cells greatly depends on their niche, and APCs being its most essential component. They include B-cells, macrophages, and dendritic cells. The last is considered as the most potent antigen-presenting cell type [31]. A role of APCs in T-cell functioning is hardly to be overestimated—they regulate activation and differentiation of T cells, shape the TCR repertoire, and assist in the cessation of unimportant immune response. Interactions of APCs with T-cells include TCR-major histocompatibility complex coupling, a contact through an array of surface molecules (adhesion, co-stimulatory, and co-inhibitory molecules), and expression of multiple soluble molecules (interleukins and cytokines).

To determine the effect of heterochronic parabiosis on APC function, we have chosen a model of PHA-mediated T-cell stimulation in the presence of total population of either $CD11c^+$ splenic dendritic cells or macrophages. During this test, T-cells are stimulated via binding of PHA. This way of T-cell stimulation is simple, reliable, and physiological instrument of measuring T-cell antigen-induced proliferation because it mimics the binding of antigen with T-cell receptor [31].

We observed the impairment of $CD11c^+$ DCs for maintaining the proliferation of young T-cells in the group of young heterochronic parabionts (**Figure 4C**).

It has been shown that the ability of splenic $CD11c^+$ dendritic cells to affect the proliferation of autologous T-cells varies slightly between young heterochronic and isochronic parabionts. But these changes are more evident in the fast-renewing population of splenic macrophages. We demonstrated decreased proliferative response of T-cells from young heterochronic parabionts when they were stimulated in vitro in the presence of macrophage-rich population of autologous splenocytes. Also, during stimulation in vitro in the presence of autologous macrophages, T-cells from young heterochronic parabionts had a lower expression of NFκB p65 on early stages of stimulation (2 h) and a higher expression of IκBα on later stages (18 h) of stimulation when compared with T-cells from young isochronic parabionts. Observed data indicate the induction of negative changes in functions of macrophage-rich population of splenocytes during heterochronic parabiosis [33].

Summarizing, immune system aging has an extremely complex mechanism, the implementation of which involved various cells, organs, and blood factors. Age-related changes give rise to changes in the properties of hematopoietic stem cells, disruption of migration routes, and differentiation mechanisms of immunocompetent T-cells, which ultimately leads to the disruption of T-cell subpopulations of lymphoid organs and their dysfunctions. Attempts to replace the old cells by young ones do not lead to the rejuvenation of the immune system. On the contrary, all the young hematopoietic stem or immune cells that were differentiated in the old organism very quickly become "old" both in its phenotype and on its functional characteristics. One of the main reasons for these changes is the microenvironment of lymphoid organs, where there is a differentiation and proliferation of HSCs and naïve T-cells. DCs, macrophages, fibroblasts, etc. are those cells which form the stroma of lymphoid organs (or lymphoid niche), and have a significant impact on the differentiation of HSCs or naïve T-cells, such as via the co-stimulatory molecules on the cell surface, as via cytokine production. And the development of approaches to the correction of age-related changes of these cell types, which form niche lymphoid organs, may help restore the age-related immune system dysfunctions in the future.

Acknowledgements

The authors are grateful to the Institute of Biology of Aging (Moscow, Russia) for supporting this work.

http://dx.doi.org/10.5772/64046

Author details

Iryna Pishel[1*] and Gennadij Butenko[2]

*Address all correspondence to: iryna.pishel@gmail.com

1 Leader Scientific Researcher, Laboratory of Pathophysiology and Immunology, D. F. Chebotaryov State Institute of Gerontology NAMS of Ukraine, Kyiv, Ukraine

2 Head of the Laboratory of Pathophysiology and Immunology, D. F. Chebotaryov State Institute of Gerontology NAMS of Ukraine, Kyiv, Ukraine

References

[1] Pawelec G, Hirokawa K, Fülöp T. Altered T cell signalling in ageing. Mech Ageing Dev. 2001;122:1613–1637. DOI:10.1016/S0047-6374(01)00290-1

[2] Caruso C, Buffa S, Candore G, Colonna-Romano G, Dunn-Walters D, Kipling D, Pawelec G. Mechanisms of immunosenescence. Immun Ageing. 2009;6:10. DOI: 10.1186/1742-4933-6-10

[3] Iscove NN, Nawa K. Hematopoietic stem cells expand during serial transplantation in vivo without apparent exhaustion. Curr Biol. 1997;7:805–808. DOI:10.1016/S0960-9822(06)00341-1

[4] Rossi DJ, Bryder D, Zahn JM, et al. Cell intrinsic alterations underlie hematopoietic stem cell aging. Proc Natl Acad Sci USA. 2005;102:9194–9199. DOI: 10.1073/pnas.0503280102

[5] Linton PJ, Dorshkind K. Age-related changes in lymphocyte development and function. Nat Immunol. 2004;5:133–139. DOI:10.1038/ni1033

[6] Wahlestedt M, Norddahl GL, Sten G, et al. An epigenetic component of hematopoietic stem cell aging amenable to reprogramming into a young state. Blood. 2013;121:4257–4264. DOI:10.1182/blood-2012-11-469080

[7] Dykstra B, Olthof S, Schreuder J, et al. Clonal analysis reveals multiple functional defects of aged murine hematopoietic stem cells. J Exp Med. 2011;208:2691–2703. DOI: 10.1084/jem.20111490

[8] Sambandam A, Bell JJ, Schwarz BA, Zediak VP, Chi AW, Zlotoff DA, Krishnamoorthy SL, Burg JM, Bhandoola A. Progenitor migration to the thymus and T cell lineage commitment. Immunol Res. 2008;42(1–3):65–74. DOI:10.1007/s12026-008-8035-z

[9] Moro-García MA, Alonso-Arias R, López-Larrea C. When aging reaches CD4+ T-cells: phenotypic and functional changes. Front Immunol. 2013;4:107. DOI:10.3389/fimmu.2013.00107

[10] Agrawal A, Agrawal S, Tay J, Gupta S. Biology of dendritic cells in aging. J Clin Immunol. 2008;28:14–20. Available from: http://link.springer.com/article/10.1007%2Fs10875-007-9127-6.

[11] Stout RD, Suttles J. Immunosenescence and macrophage functional plasticity: dysregulation of macrophage function by age-associated microenvironmental changes. Immunol Rev. 2005;205:60–71. DOI:10.1111/j.0105-2896.2005.00260.x

[12] Sidorenko AV, Gubrii IB, Andrianova LF, Maksiuk TV, Butenko GM. Functional rearrangement of lymphohemopoietic system in heterochronically parabiosed mice. Mech Ageing Dev. 1986;36:41–56. DOI:10.1016/0047-6374(86)90137-5

[13] Butenko GM, Gubrii IB. Inhibition of the immune responses of young adult CBA mice due to parabiosis with their old partners. Exp Geront. 1980;15:605–610. DOI:10.1016/0531-5565(80)90012-1

[14] Deyl Z, Butenko GM, Hausmann J, Novakova M, Macek K. Increased glycation and pigmentation of collagen in aged and young parabiotic rats and mice. Mech Ageing Dev. 1990;55:39–47. DOI:10.1016/0047-6374(90)90104-N

[15] Hirokawa K, Utsuyama M. Combined grafting of bone marrow and thymus, and sequential multiple thymus graftings in various strains of mice. The effect on immune functions and life span. Mech Ageing Dev. 1989;49(1):49–60. DOI:10.1016/0047-6374(89)90067-5

[16] Bunster E, Meyer RK. An improved method of parabiosis. Anat Rec. 1933;57:339–343. DOI:10.1002/ar.1090570404

[17] Barisic-Dujmovic T, Boban I, Clark SH. Fibroblasts/myofibroblasts that participate in cutaneous wound healing are not derived from circulating progenitor cells. J Cell Physiol. 2010;222:703–712. DOI:10.1002/jcp.21997

[18] Abe S, Boyer C, Liu X, Wen FQ, Kobayashi T, Fang Q, Wang X, Hashimoto M, Sharp JG, Rennard SI. Cells derived from the circulation contribute to the repair of lung injury. Am J Respir Crit Care Med. 2004;170:1158–1163. DOI:10.1164/rccm.200307-908OC

[19] Pietramaggiori G, Scherer SS, Alperovich M, Chen B, Orgill DP, Wagers AJ. Improved cutaneous healing in diabetic mice exposed to healthy peripheral circulation. J Investig Dermatol. 2009;129:2265–2274. DOI:10.1038/jid.2009.60

[20] Goldman DC, Bailey AS, Pfaffle DL, Al Masri A, Christian JL, Fleming WH. BMP4 regulates the hematopoietic stem cell niche. Blood. 2009;114:4393–4401. DOI:10.1182/blood-2009-02-206433

[21] Aicher A, Rentsch M, Sasaki K, Ellwart JW, Fandrich F, Siebert R, Cooke JP, Dimmeler S, Heeschen C. Nonbone marrow-derived circulating progenitor cells contribute to

postnatal neovascularization following tissue ischemia. Circ Res. 2007;100:581–589. DOI:10.1161/01.RES.0000259562.63718.35

[22] Purhonen S, Palm J, Rossi D, Kaskenpaa N, Rajantie I, Yla-Herttuala S, Alitalo K, Weissman IL, Salven P. Bone marrow-derived circulating endothelial precursors do not contribute to vascular endothelium and are not needed for tumor growth. Proc Natl Acad Sci USA. 2008;105:6620–6625. DOI:10.1073/pnas.0710516105

[23] Hirokawa K, Utsuyama M, Kobayashi S. Hypothalamic control of development and aging of the thymus. Mech Ageing Dev. 1998;100:177–185. DOI:10.1016/S0047-6374(97)00135-8

[24] Pishel I, Shytikov D, Orlova T, Peregudov A, Artyuhov I, Butenko G. Accelerated aging versus rejuvenation of the immune system in heterochronic parabiosis. Rejuvenation Res. 2012;15:239–248. DOI:10.1089/rej.2012.1331

[25] Wakikawa A, Utsuyama M, Hirokawa K. Altered expression of various receptors on T cells in young and old mice after mitogenic stimulation: a flow cytometric analysis. Mech Ageing Dev. 1997;94:113–122. DOI:10.1016/S0047-6374(97)01880-0

[26] Parretta E, Cassese G, Santoni A, Guardiola J, Vecchio A, Di Rosa F. Kinetics of in vivo proliferation and death of memory and naive CD8 T cells: parameter estimation based on 5-bromo-2-deoxyuridine incorporation in spleen, lymph nodes, and bone marrow. J Immunol. 2008;180:7230–7239. DOI:10.4049/?jimmunol.180.11.7230

[27] Blais MÈ, Brochu S, Giroux M, Bèlanger MP, Dulude G, Sèkaly RP, Perreault C. Why T cells of thymic versus extrathymic origin are functionally different. J Immunol. 2008;180:2299–2312. DOI:10.4049/?jimmunol.180.4.2299

[28] Cheung KP, Yang E, Goldrath AW. Memory-like CD8+ T cells generated during homeostatic proliferation defer to antigen-experienced memory cells. J Immunol. 2009;183:3364–3372. DOI:10.4049/jimmunol.0900641

[29] Zhang X, Fujii H, Kishimoto H, LeRoy E, Surh CD, Sprent J. Aging leads to disturbed homeostasis of memory phenotype CD8+ Cells. J Exp Med. 2002;195:283–293. DOI: 10.1084/jem.20011267

[30] Cools N, Ponsaerts P, Van Tendeloo VF, Berneman ZN. Balancing between immunity and tolerance: an interplay between dendritic cells, regulatory T cells, and effector T cells. J Leukoc Biol. 2007;82:1365–1374. DOI:10.1189/jlb.0307166

[31] Linehan E, Fitzgerald DC. Ageing and the immune system: focus on macrophages. Eur J Microbiol Immunol (Bp). 2015;5(1):14–24. DOI:10.1556/EUJMI-D-14-00035

[32] Kruisbeek AM, Shevach E, Thornton AM. Proliferative assays for T cell function. Curr Protoco Immunol. 2004;60:III:3.12:3.12.1–3.12.20. DOI:10.1002/0471142735.im0312s60

[33] Shytikov DW, Shkumat MS, Yankova TM, Peregudov AG, Artyuhov IV, Pishel IM. Splenic Niche cells from young heterochronic parabionts have decreased capability to

amplify T-cell proliferation in vitro. Am J BioSci. 2015;3(2):46–54. DOI:10.11648/j.ajbio.20150302.14

[34] Tsukamoto H, Clise-Dwyer K, Huston GE, Duso DK, Buck AL, Johnson LL, et al. Age-associated increase in lifespan of naive CD4 T cells contributes to T-cell homeostasis but facilitates development of functional defects. Proc Natl Acad Sci USA. 2009;106:18333–18338. DOI:10.1073/pnas.0910139106

Chapter 6

New Perspectives in the Diagnosis of Mild Cognitive Impairment and Alzheimer's Disease: Novel Uses of Biomarkers

Judit Subirana-Mirete

Additional information is available at the end of the chapter

http://dx.doi.org/10.5772/64322

Abstract

Criteria for the diagnosis of Alzheimer's disease were established in 1984 by the National Institute of Neurological and Communicative Disorders and Stroke (NINCDS) and the Alzheimer's Disease and Related Disorders Association (ADRDA). Commonly used since their implementation, these criteria are becoming obsolete for everyday practice, and a review is being claimed. Three groups of experts consisting of renowned experts from the National Institute on Aging (NIA) and the Alzheimer's Association proposed a set of recommendations to modify the criteria in this field of research. Two notable differences from the initial criteria were included: the incorporation of biomarkers and the formalization of different disease stages in the diagnostic criteria. From now on, mild cognitive impairment is incorporated in the diagnosis as another stage of dementia. However, the new criteria are still under revision and are currently of use for research purposes with the aim to get the definitive modification for the clinical criteria. This chapter presents the main developments in research concerning Alzheimer's disease and mild cognitive impairment to define these new research criteria.

Keywords: Alzheimer's disease, mild cognitive impairment, biomarkers, neuropsychology, dementia

1. Introduction

The concept of dementia makes us instantly think about a set of characteristic symptoms and the resulting repercussions for patients and their families. The objective of this chapter is to update our ideas about Alzheimer's disease and get to know the beginning and evolution of the construct of mild cognitive impairment, as well as the new advances in genetics and biomarkers that, in not such a distant future, will be of common use in the diagnosis of cognitive impairment.

The Greeks were the first to study mental disorders from a scientific point of view by separating the study of mind from religion. The existence of dementia has been known since the times of Hippocrates (460–370 BC), although throughout history, it has been given different names: paranoia, idiocy, senility, senile psychosis, and so on. But it will not be until 1906 that Alois Alzheimer first described the disease that would be named after him and which has made history worldwide [1].

From Dr. Alois Alzheimer's first patient, Auguste D., until the current description and definition of the disease, more than a century has passed and many research studies have been carried out on it. Initially, it was considered to be a condition particular to young patients, and so it was given the name of presenile dementia. However, the progressive increase in life expectancy left uncovered that the symptoms present in Auguste D. were also found in older population, thus leading to a new approach to the disease. But it was not until the 1970s that the disease described by Alzheimer started to be a focus of attention. The real story of the concept of dementia and Alzheimer's disease can be consulted in different texts of reference [1–3].

Recently, knowledge on dementia in general and on Alzheimer's disease in particular has been remarkably expanded. The diagnostic process for Alzheimer's disease has benefitted from widely accepted consensus protocols [4]. Nevertheless, the clinical heterogeneity of this disease (age of onset, type of impairment, or the disease's progression pace) makes diagnosis extremely difficult.

2. Diagnosis of Alzheimer's disease

Alzheimer's disease is a neurodegenerative condition of insidious onset and progressive evolution, characterized by loss of memory and other cognitive functions, and by a set of noncognitive symptoms, among which depressive or psychotic-related symptoms and behaviour disorders stand out. Among the main neuropsychological features of this disease, we can point at the progressive impairment of memory and language, the decline in visuospatial and motor capacities, and the disruption of executive functions such as the capacity for abstraction and reasoning [5, 6].

The criteria for the clinical diagnosis of Alzheimer's disease were defined in 1984 by the National Institute of Neurological and Communicative Disorders (NINCD) and the Alzheimer's Disease and Related-Disorders Association (ADRDA). These criteria are based on the idea that Alzheimer's disease is a single clinicopathological entity [7], thus advocating that Alzheimer's disease always has a close correlation between clinical symptoms and their pathological basis; in most cases, it was thought that the typical anatomopathological presentation already described in 1910 and based on the presence of senile plaques, neurofibrillary tangles and cerebral arteriosclerotic changes [8] would be found at autopsy. Following this idea, the basic lines for the development of the disease were, in 1984, as follows:

1. The underlying pathology of Alzheimer's disease and clinical symptoms was developed concurrently.

2. Patients either had completely developed Alzheimer's disease symptoms (in this case, then, they clearly had a dementia), or they were free of this pathology and, therefore, had no dementia at all (at least no Alzheimer-like dementia as later identified).

Thus, 1984 criteria required the presence of cognitive impairment and dementia to be confirmed by neuropsychological assessment in order to establish the diagnosis of possible or probable Alzheimer's disease, although histopathological confirmation was still needed for a final diagnosis (via autopsy or biopsy) (see **Table 1**).

NINCDS-ADRDA (1984) criteria for the clinical diagnosis of Alzheimer's disease	
Diagnostic criteria for probable Alzheimer's disease: Presence of dementia: - Established by clinical examination - Documented by the Mini-Mental Cognitive Examination Test, Blessed Dementia Scale or similar - Confirmed by neuropsychological tests - Deficits in two or more areas of cognition - Progressive worsening of memory and other cognitive functions - No disturbance of consciousness - Onset between ages 40 and 90 - Absence of systemic disorders or other brain disease that could cause dementia	**Diagnostic criteria for possible Alzheimer's disease:** - Dementia syndrome in the absence of other causes and in the presence of variations in the onset, in the presentation, or in the clinical course - Presence of another systemic or brain disorder sufficient to produce dementia, which is not considered to be *the* cause of the dementia - Presence of a single, progressive severe cognitive deficit
Criteria that support the diagnosis of probable Alzheimer's disease: - Progressive deterioration of specific cognitive functions (e.g., language, motor skills, perception - Impaired activities of daily living (ADL) and altered patterns of behaviour - Family history of similar disorders - Consistency in analytic results (lumbar puncture, EEG, CT)	**Diagnostic criteria for definite Alzheimer's disease:** - Meeting the clinical criteria for probable Alzheimer's disease with histopathologic evidence
Features nonconsistent with the diagnosis of Alzheimer's disease. Sudden onset - Focal neurologic signs - Seizures or early gait disturbances	

Source: Adapted from Carrasco [21].

Table 1. Criteria for the diagnosis of Alzheimer's disease.

Some aspects of these criteria have been set aside by new research and daily clinical practice has also pointed at ideas to be revised. The pathological histology present in Alzheimer's disease can also be found in a wide set of alternative clinical conditions [9, 10], from patients without cognitive symptoms to patients with mild cognitive impairment (MCI) or other types of impairment. Therefore, the initial concept of Alzheimer's disease has to be less restrictive than that developed in 1984.

The capacity to recognize some clinical symptoms in other disorders with a similar development as in Alzheimer's disease was limited two decades ago, thus resulting in diagnostic confusions. In this respect, for example, reversible systemic disorders such as vitamin B12 deficiency, which may have similar symptoms to a dementia, were not taken into consideration [11]. Although frontotemporal dementia was considered to be an entity, others such as Lewy body dementia or vascular dementia were not taken into account [12]. Likewise, the concept of aphasia linked to neurodegenerative disorders, despite being described some years before the NINCDS-ADRDA criteria [13], was not fully developed until two decades later [14].

The implication that memory impairment must always be considered as the primary cognitive deficit for the diagnosis of Alzheimer's disease is also being put into doubt, as clinical experience has showed that Alzheimer's disease may be developed in a nonamnesic way [15]. Clinical experience has also pointed at the need to revise cut-off points by age for the diagnosis, as age-related pathologies such as dementia are more and more frequent due to the overageing of population. Finally, the inclusion of new results from neuroimaging exploration and biomarker clinical analysis in the new criteria will allow us to get to know the individual characteristics of every cognitive impairment from an integral approach of the same construct.

Since the establishment of the NINCDS-ADRDA criteria 32 years ago, it has been proved that Alzheimer's disease underlying pathology and clinical symptoms are not always present concurrently, thus dismissing one of the main assumptions of the 1984 diagnostic criteria. Research has evolved remarkably since then and, among other events, it has been identified, for example, that in the absence of any apparent symptom, there can be a wide pathological presentation (particularly of amyloid plaques) [16, 17].

Knowledge about the neuropathology of Alzheimer's disease has been expanded in the last 25 years of the twentieth century; new sets of diagnostic criteria to establish a diagnosis of this disease from its neuropathological basis have been developed and applied more or less successfully. Among others, we have to consider those by the National Institute on Aging (NIA) [18], those by the Consortium to Establish a Registry for Alzheimer's Disease (CERAD) [19], and those by the NIA-Reagan Institute [20]. There are no basic differences among these three classifications; they all stand out the need to carry out an inclusive diagnosis, establish the priority for the cognitive diagnosis—with special emphasis on memory—and consider other noncognitive or psychiatric symptoms to be "accessory" [21]. These approaches present two main problems: first, they downplay cognitive symptoms, as they only focus on amnesic manifestations, with the other cognitive functions and psychopathological impairments being left in the background; second, they are limited by the inability to categorize certain symptoms present in this kind of dementia [22]. Nevertheless, there are two main research aspects that have evolved from the very first description of this disease: using biomarkers and formally establishing different stages for the disease. Literature on mild cognitive impairment has exponentially increased since the 1990s in order to document the gradual impairment of cognitive functions preceding the point when there is a significant interference with activities of daily living [23]. As previously mentioned, the 1984 criteria did not consider cognitive impairment that does not reach the dementia threshold, thus passing over that the Alzheimer's disease underlying pathology slowly develops for years—or even decades—before there is a clinical manifestation of the disease.

3. Mild cognitive impairment

Different nosological entities have been defined in order to characterize cognitive impairment processes that represent an intermediate stage between cognitive decline observed in the ageing process and changes that meet the criteria for the diagnosis of dementia [24]. The most used concept is that of "mild cognitive impairment" (MCI) coined by Petersen et al. [25], although initially described by Flicker et al. [26] according to Reisberg's Global Deterioration Scale [27].

MCI is a syndrome that shows up as a cognitive dysfunction greater than expected for the patient's age and cultural and educational level, that develops without major interferences in activities of daily living and does not meet criteria for dementia [25, 28]. The main diagnostic difference between Alzheimer's disease and mild cognitive impairment lies in the degree of interference in the patient's capacity to develop daily work or regular tasks. This is, unavoidably, a determination to be carried out by an expert on the basis of individual circumstances and the description of daily routines obtained by both the patient and a close informant. For a further development of this differential diagnosis, please see Albert et al. [29].

The definition in Petersen [21] describes MCI as a degenerative process that precedes dementia —on the basis of the *cognitive continuum* construct (**Figure 1**), where the main deficit concerns memory and the other cognitive functions seem to be stable. Later studies have expanded the MCI construct by describing different subtypes not only limited to amnestic symptoms [30].

Nelson and O'Connor [31] described, through postmortem histopathological studies with MCI patients, that a wide majority of cases evolved to a process of dementia, although a small percentage did not. These results put into question the assumption that MCI may always be considered as an initial stage of Alzheimer's disease.

As we get closer to the definition of the earliest stages of cognitive impairment, the dissociation between the connotations of the concept of early Alzheimer's disease and MCI is more obvious. It is becoming clearer and clearer that both Alzheimer's disease pathophysiological process and symptoms are better explained as a continuum (linking both Alzheimer's disease and MCI at the same time), as these processes can concurrently evolve and even overlap in time [32]. Hence the need to revise both constructs further.

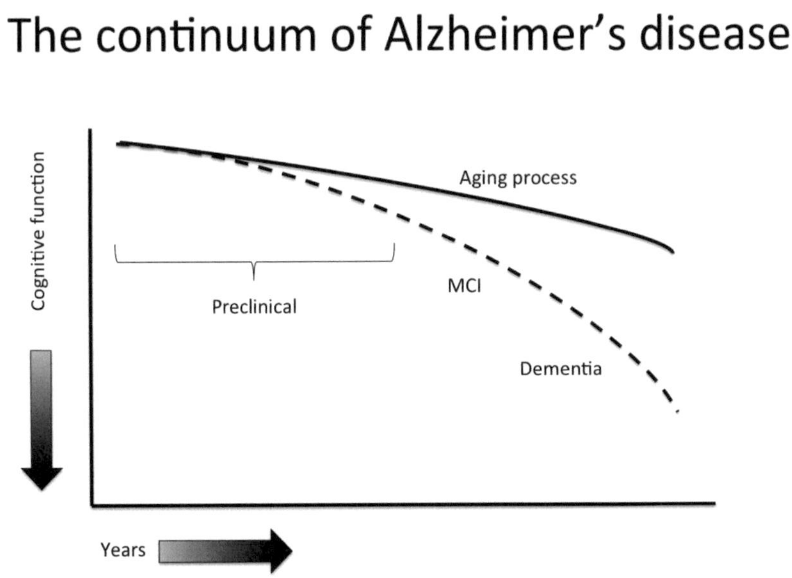

Figure 1. Model of cognitive continuum. Adapted from Sperling et al. [32].

Although some agreement has been reached in the last few years, the current MCI diagnosis is complex as there are no precise and standardized criteria with general consensus. As main characteristics, we can stand out the complaints about memory loss from the beginning of the process, reported either by an informant or by the patients themselves. Patients often report other symptoms, such as difficulties to find needed words, loss of personal objects, disorientation, or loss of continuity in usual tasks, for example, in a conversation [31].

There have been attempts to formalize these clinical observations as diagnostic criteria. We can stand out those by the Study Group on Dementia and Behavioral Disorders of the Spanish Society of Neurology [33] or those by Mayo Clinic [25] that correspond to the amnestic subtype only. Also worth highlighting are those by the International Psychogeriatric Association (IPA) [34], described in **Table 2**.

Despite the efforts to agree on diagnostic criteria for MCI, there are still some difficulties deriving, in many cases, from conceptual limitations of the nosological entity itself [24]. Since the Montreal Consensus [35], criteria became more flexible, with the inclusion, for instance, not only of patients in a cognitive normality dementia transition stage but also very prevalent intermediate conditions secondary to other aetiologies (e.g., vascular dementia) or other conditions, also very frequent, such as those secondary to mood disorders [36].

One of the facts that has always been an object of attention is the relationship between MCI and dementia, in particular, Alzheimer's disease [30, 37]. A recently published study [38] reports the prevalence for mild cognitive impairment between 3 and 42% depending on the construct. We should remember now that, before Petersen et al.'s definition of MCI [25], other constructs had been considered such as age-associated memory impairment (AAMI) [27] or cognitive impairment no dementia (CIND) [39]. In particular, according to Ward's study,

AAMI prevalence is between 3.6 and 38.4%; the prevalence for CIND ranges between a bit more than 5 and 35.9%, whereas studies using the concept of MCI (as described by Petersen) show population prevalence between 3 and 42%. Moreover, if we consider that MCI patients have a three times higher risk to develop Alzheimer's disease in a period of 4.5 years after diagnosis [40], the need for some criteria that are agreed upon, global and useful for the diagnosis of cognitive impairment in all of its stages, from onset to more serious stages, becomes particularly important.

Diagnostic criteria according to the International Psychogeriatric Association (IPA) and World Health Organization (WHO)
1. No age restriction
2. Decline of cognitive function reported by patient or informant
3. Decline is gradual and present for at least 6 months
4. Deterioration in any major cognitive domain: - Memory and learning - Attention and concentration - Language - Thinking - Visuospatial functioning
5. Lower scores in mental state evaluations or neuropsychological tests, a standard deviation below the mean value of a control group
6. No presence of brain processes, either systemic or psychiatric, that can account for the impairment

Source: Adapted from Sánchez-Rodríguez and Torrellas-Morales [28].

Table 2. IPA criteria.

Since 2009 there has been a consensus among the main research centres, that diagnostic criteria for Alzheimer's disease, as well as those for dementia and mild cognitive impairment, should be revised. For this reason, the National Institute on Aging (NIA), together with the Alzheimer's Association, sponsored a deep revision of criteria, thus establishing a revision of old criteria by three independent groups of experts. The first group undertook to establish and describe diagnostic criteria for dementia and Alzheimer's disease; the second group focused on the symptomatic stage prior to Alzheimer-like dementia; finally, the third group dealt with the asymptomatic stage prior to dementia and mild cognitive impairment. The recommendations of the three groups were presented at the 2010 International Conference on Alzheimer's Disease and later published [41]. This new proposal of criteria has integrated research on dementia, MCI, and Alzheimer's disease carried out in the last 25 years of the twentieth century. In particular, the inclusion of genetic breakthroughs, biomarkers, and final formalization of the different stages in the development of dementia are worth standing out.

4. New advances in research

The role of genetics in the diagnosis of the different types of cognitive impairment is more and more active and important. At present, there is no doubt about the existence of genetic risk factors to develop Alzheimer's disease, as some genes have been identified that are not only responsible for the genetically pure forms of the disease but also some sporadic and late-onset forms [42].

Although the most important risk factor related to Alzheimer's disease is the ageing process of the patient, the second risk factor is the family history of the disease. Thus, Alzheimer's disease is a complex pathology with a clear genetic component. Up to now, three genes have been found to be responsible for early onset familial Alzheimer's disease: the gene for amyloid beta precursor protein (APP), the gene for presenilin-1 (PS1), and the gene for presenilin-2 (PS2). Taking this into account, if the predominant autosomal form of Alzheimer's disease is present in a patient with MCI, then this MCI is more likely to be a prodrome of early onset Alzheimer's disease [43].

But not only is early onset Alzheimer's disease linked to genetic influence. Approximately, 40% of diagnosed individuals have a family history of the disease, and epidemiological studies show that the risk of developing the disease if a first-degree relative already has it is between two and three times higher than that of general population [44]. The genetic component of late-onset Alzheimer's disease has been targeted in many studies, but at the moment only a genetic component, APOE, has been considered as a risk factor associated with the disease [43]. Thus, up to now, the presence of one or two ε4 alleles in the gene for apolipoprotein E (APOE) has been the only genetic variation widely accepted as a risk factor to develop late-onset Alzheimer's disease, whereas the presence of the ε2 allele would have the opposite effect [45]. Evidence suggests, then, that an individual meeting clinical, cognitive, and etiological criteria for MCI and carrier of the ε4 allele of the APOE gene is more likely to progress towards developing Alzheimer's disease, eventually, than any other individual without this genetic characteristic.

Genetic research has also allowed us to know that the molecular mechanisms that start Alzheimer's disease, both clinically and pathologically, correspond to a metabolic disorder of amyloid beta (Aβ) [46]. A key point is the concept according to which some usually soluble neuronal proteins can misfold and aggregate, for instance, in neurofibrillary tangles, thus producing high levels of cell cytotoxicity [47]. Recent data suggest that although familial Alzheimer's disease is characterized by Aβ overproduction, sporadic late-onset forms are characterized by a decrease in Aβ recycling capacity. And Aβ traffic is controlled by APOE, so the genetic data available at the moment overwhelmingly point at the amyloid cascade hypothesis as the starter of the cognitive impairment process [48].

To facilitate the theoretical discussion of the MCI construct as a preclinical stage of Alzheimer's disease, the group revising the criteria [32] proposed a theoretical model to explain the relationship between cognitive decline and the basic pathophysiology of Alzheimer's disease (see **Figure 2**). As will be seen later, genetic factors are not the only determinants in the development and progression of mild cognitive impairment, as other risk factors, such as vascular factors or the history of personal development, as well as environmental factors and cognitive reserve, which can positively influence the development of cognitive symptoms of decline, also have to be considered.

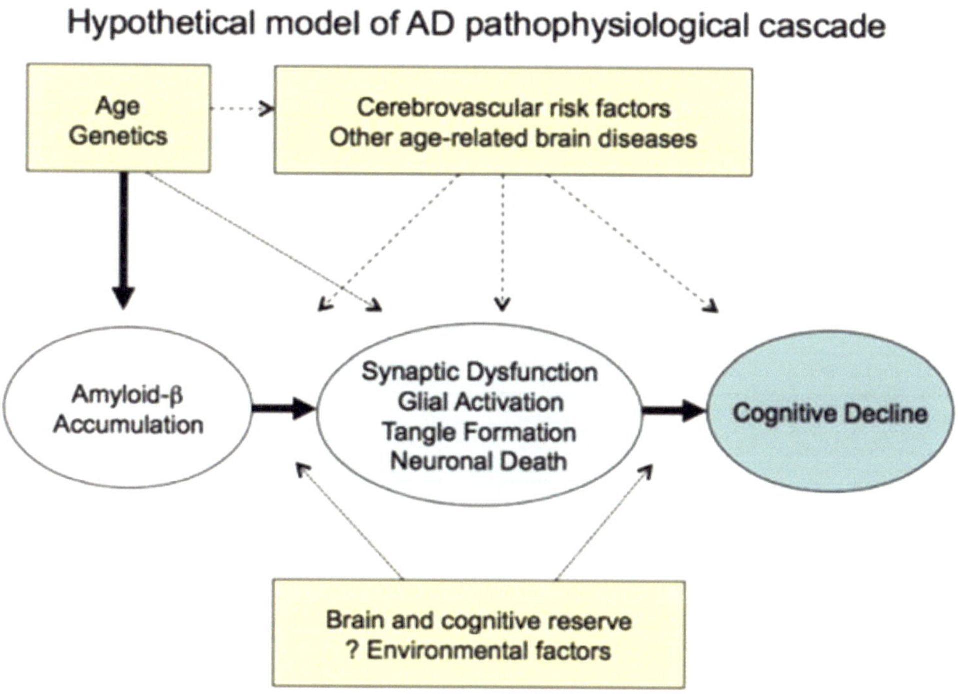

Figure 2. Relationship between cognitive decline and the basic pathophysiology of Alzheimer's disease. Based on Sperling et al. [32].

Another remarkable difference between the 1984 criteria and those revised in 2011 is the incorporation of biomarkers to diagnose cognitive impairment. Biomarkers are physiological, biochemical, or anatomic parameters that are measured in vivo and that reflect specific characteristics of pathophysiological processes related to a disease; in this case, MCI or Alzheimer's disease. It is important to incorporate new knowledge on biomarkers into the diagnostic framework of these diseases, as, on the one hand, they provide us with greater support when establishing the etiological bases of the cognitive decline process and thus allow us to better choose the intervention to follow when there are effective specific treatments; on the other hand, they allow us to determine the probability of the cognitive and functional progression of impairment towards a more serious stage of MCI or towards dementia, as well as the possibility that this progression develops in a defined period of time [29].

There are many biomarkers. Nevertheless, after a long and thorough study of the main markers, the study groups selected only two categories of biomarkers to be included in their recommendations. These are the biomarkers related to Aβ and the biomarkers reflecting neuronal injury [29].

The amyloid plaques (or senile plaques) are one of the most characteristic features of Alzheimer's disease and, therefore, those biomarkers that can detect and quantify Aβ protein or tau protein accumulated in brain tissue are vitally important for the pathological diagnosis of the disease and its precursors [49]. Aβ deposition markers include both measurements of the level of $A\beta_{42}$ in cerebrospinal fluid (CSF) as evidence of deposition via positron emission tomography (PET) imaging by using a variety of specific binding agents [50]. Tau protein accumulation markers can be obtained through measurements via CSF.

Among neuronal injury markers, there is a series of structural and functional measures, described in **Table 3**, together with Aβ biomarkers.

Biomarkers for the diagnosis of cognitive impairment
Biomarkers of Aβ deposition - CSF $A\beta_{42}$ - PET amyloid imaging
Biomarkers of neuronal injury - CSF tau/phosphorylated-tau - Hippocampal volume or medial temporal atrophy by volumetric measures - Rate of brain atrophy - FDG-PET imaging - SPECT perfusion measures *Other non-validated measures*: fMRI activation studies, resting BOLD functional connectivity, MRI perfusion, MR spectroscopy, and diffusion tensor imaging.

Abbreviations: CSF, cerebrospinal fluid; PET, positron emission tomography; FDG, fluorodeoxyglucose; SPECT, single photon emission tomography; fMRI, functional magnetic resonance imaging; BOLD, blood oxygen level-dependent; MR, magnetic resonance.
Adapted from Albert et al. [29].

Table 3. Biomarkers for clinical diagnosis.

Among the potential uses of biomarkers, there is the identification of people in the preclinical stages of the disease or the reduction in the heterogeneity of the disease in clinical trials. However, not all biomarkers are valid as indirect assessment criteria, as they can be difficult to validate and require different levels of validation depending on their expected use. In this respect, although the presence of high levels of tau protein is clearly associated with the pathophysiological process of Alzheimer's disease, changes in tau and phosphorylated-tau (p-Tau) are not exclusive to Alzheimer's disease and can also reflect more general neuronal and synaptic damage. The same can be said of Aβ depositions, as they are not exclusive to Alzheimer's disease. This is one of the main limitations of these biomarkers [51]. No conclusive determination has been reached either concerning whether the quantitative measure of these biomarkers provides us with more information than the dichotomous assessment (presence/absence; positive/negative). Nevertheless, the combination of both types of measures points

http://dx.doi.org/10.5772/64322

at the higher probability that the pathophysiological process of the disease is the etiological base of underlying changes [29].

One of the main drawbacks in Alzheimer's disease research is that the symptoms of the disease appear after significant neuronal loss. The objective of current research with biomarkers is to manage to prevent this loss before the final emergence of symptoms, in order to develop really efficient treatments against this disease, as current medication can only provide patients with short-term improvements of their cognitive function [52].

5. New criteria for research on mild cognitive impairment and Alzheimer's disease

After thoroughly analysing the background and revising the main research studies carried out at the epidemiological, neuropsychological, genetic levels, and with biomarkers, the group of experts of the National Institute on Aging and the Alzheimer's Association proposed a working framework (**Figure 3**) to provide specialists, and the scientific world in general, with a specific and common language to move towards the knowledge of the preclinical and clinical stages of Alzheimer's disease.

The objective of the group of experts is to contribute with some operational research criteria in order to help select future target groups at risk of developing Alzheimer's disease, by considering the presence of Aβ biomarkers (either in isolation or in combination with other neurodegeneration markers). We have to consider that, at the moment, the use of these new criteria is for research only and that an inappropriate use in other fields may lead to wrong results and misinterpretations, as so far these criteria are still under revision.

These new criteria are based on the assumption that Alzheimer's disease is characterized by a sequence of biological events that begin much before the clinical symptoms of the disease appear. Considering the genetic evidence, the hypothesis of Aβ accumulation in a first stage of amyloidosis, which would be the first moment when cognitive impairment can be measured, is gaining strength. This first stage occurs before any other symptomatic manifestation and, therefore, would allow for a first diagnosis, which would indicate that a still indefinable process has started. At the same time, the new criteria acknowledge that the preclinical stages of Alzheimer's disease represent a continuum, including those cases that will never go beyond stage 1 or 2. The presence of one or two biomarkers, once the MCI stage has been reached, would indicate that an individual is experiencing a neurodegenerative process that in further stages will be defined.

As the group of experts highlights in their conclusions [32], at the moment, these criteria are to be used only in research and have no diagnostic utility; the objective of the new criteria is to allow researchers to better characterize the biological sequence that triggers Alzheimer's disease from the first moments. Therefore, these criteria have to facilitate the standardization of data collection in new studies, whose results will modify the very same criteria.

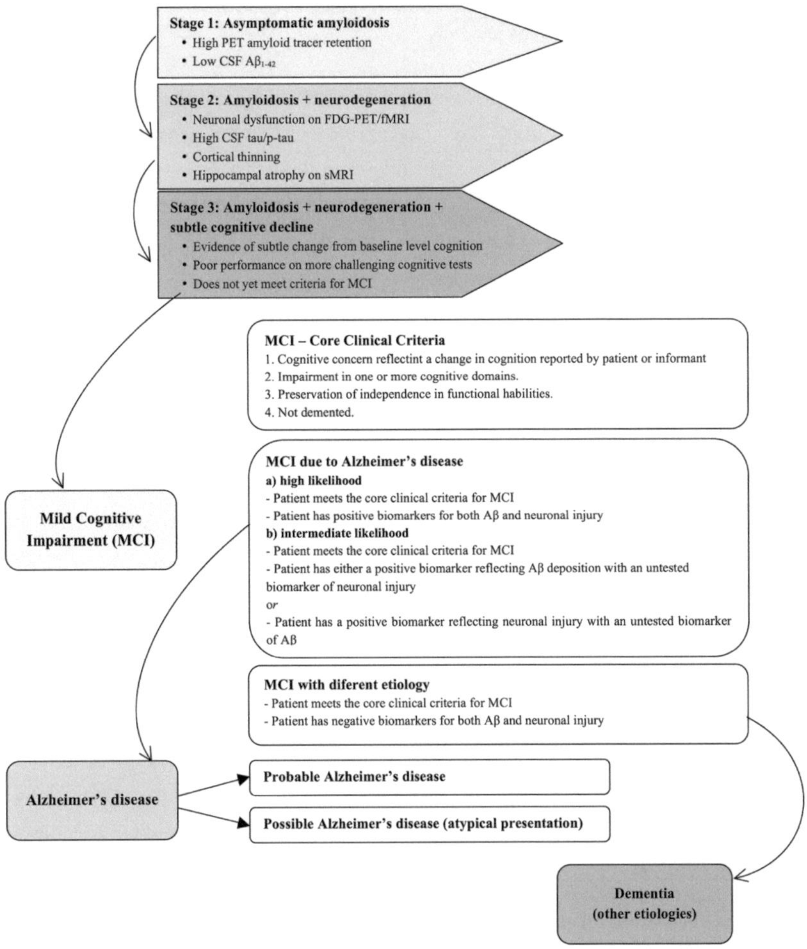

Figure 3. New proposal for research criteria for MCI and Alzheimer's disease.

6. Neuropsychological contributions to the early detection of cognitive impairment

Research has highlighted, beyond the genetic base, a series of factors that have a crucial significance in the development and course of cognitive impairment and Alzheimer's disease. There is great interest in knowing, for example, the association between two facts: cognitive impairment and metabolic and vascular alterations, such as cardiovascular diseases, high blood pressure, diabetes, or obesity, on the one hand, and the establishment and course of the disease, on the other. Understanding these relationships and obtaining data via clinical studies can help us understand that the fact of reducing risk factors associated to these pathologies may be also useful to control Alzheimer's disease. Moreover, a healthy balanced diet, physical

http://dx.doi.org/10.5772/64322

exercise, social commitment, and mentally challenging activities can help people to keep healthy as they get older [53].

With regard to environmental factors, included in the diagram of **Figure 2**, different studies show that a higher educational level, complex working activities or a socially integrated lifestyle are factors that can help to postpone the onset of clinical cognitive impairment [54, 55]. It has also been shown that physical exercise and cardiovascular activity have long-term benefits on cognition [56]. Actually, physical activity has been proved to reduce the risk of developing dementia and to improve cognition [57].

On the other hand, vascular risk factors are associated, by definition, to vascular dementia. In contrast, the relationship between vascular risk factors and the development and progression of cognitive impairment associated with Alzheimer's disease is less clear. For more than three decades, Alzheimer's disease has been described as a primary neurodegenerative disorder with scarce, or none, vascular foundation [5, 58]. Nevertheless, in the last few years, knowledge about this relationship has increased a lot and many current studies relate vascular risk factors to the pathogenesis of mild cognitive impairment and Alzheimer's disease (see De la Torre for a thorough theoretical revision [59]).

Knowledge about the risk factors of Alzheimer's disease has expanded a lot, and at present, they include not only risk factors particular to the ageing and adulthood process but also risk factors particular to all life stages. For example, perinatal conditions, brain development, growth factors, socioeconomic conditions, or cognitive reserve are factors that have been shown to have an influence on the process of developing dementia [60, 61].

The identification of prodromal neuropsychological markers in cognitive impairment is based on the idea that neuronal loss starts much earlier than clinical symptoms. For this, it is essential to clinically detect individuals in the first stages of impairment, as starting treatment in these early moments would help to maximize the impact on maintaining cognitive functions and functional skills. Hence, the importance of having adapted tests to detect cognitive impairment at early stages, as an early diagnosis of cognitive impairment at prodromal stages is still a very important objective, considering the probability that this stage will be susceptible to treatments designed both to stop and to slow down the progression of the impairment.

In summary, literature suggests that the risk of starting a process of cognitive impairment linked to Alzheimer's disease is not determined only by a genetic component or by certain risk factors in adulthood, but by the result of a complex interaction between genetic and environmental factors throughout our entire life.

In the next decades, an increase in the prevalence of Alzheimer's disease in particular and cognitive impairment in general is expected. Advances in clinical research will make the management of this disease more sophisticated. In the near future, there will be new tests to identify both people at risk of developing Alzheimer's disease and those having early symptoms of cognitive impairment. At the same time, there will be more medicines available and possibly the progression of the disease may be delayed for years. With the improvement in diagnosis and early detection of Alzheimer's disease, more people will be diagnosed at the early stages of the disease. The role of the family will be more and more crucial, as together with early diagnosis and pharmacological treatment there will be coordination of care and support functions both for patients and for carers of people with dementia. Many of these individuals will have the added value of still being there for their families, to look after children, for example, or being an important part in the ageing of the parents themselves. To improve care and support to these people, the public and private sectors have to work together to eliminate age-related barriers that reduce access to help and support services and to improve the comprehension of the unique needs of the people diagnosed with Alzheimer's disease and their environment.

Author details

Judit Subirana-Mirete

Address all correspondence to: juditsm@blanquerna.edu

Faculty of Psychology, Education and Sport Sciences Blanquerna, Ramon Llull University, Barcelona, Spain

References

[1] Maurer K, Maurer U. Alzheimer. La vida de un médico y la historia de una enfermedad [The life of a doctor and the history of a disease]. Barcelona: Díaz de Santos; 2006.

[2] Berrios, G. (2000). Historical overview. In: O'Brien J, Ames D, Burns A, editors. Dementia 2nd ed. London: Arnold; 2000, pp. 3–13.

[3] Brick KL. The history of Alzheimer's Association. Future public policy implications. In: Maurer K, Ballenger JF, editors. Concepts of Alzheimer disease. Biological, clinical and cultural perspectives. Baltimore, John Hopkins; 2000. pp. 234–239.

[4] Small G, Rabins P, Barry P, Buckholtz N, DeKosky S, Ferris S, et al. Diagnosis and treatment of Alzheimer's disease and related disorders. Consensus statement of the American Association for Geriatric Psychiatry, the Alzheimer's Association and the American Geriatrics Society. Journal of the American Medical Association. 1997; 278: 1363–1371. DOI: 10.1001/jama.278.16.1363.

[5] American Psychiatric Association. The Diagnostic and Statistical Manual of Mental Disorders. 4th edition revised. Barcelona: Elsevier-Masson; 2001.

[6] Subirana J, Crusat M, Cullell N, Cuevas R, Signo S. Demencias y enfermedad de Alzheimer [Dementia and Alzheimer's Disease]. In: Bruna O, Roig T, Puyuelo M,

Junqué C, Ruano A, editors. Rehabilitación neuropsicológica [Neuropsychological rehabilitation]. Barcelona: Elsevier, Masson; 2011. pp. 289–318.

[7] McKhann G, Drachman D, Folstein M, Katzman R, Prince D, Standlan E. Clinical Diagnosis of Alzheimer's Disease: Report of the NINCDS-ADRDA Work Group under the auspices of Department of Health and Human Services Task Force on Alzheimer's disease. Neurology. 1984; 34: 939–944.

[8] Kraepelin E. Psychiatrie: Em Lehrbuch für Studierende und Ärzte [A Textbook for Students and Doctors]. Leipzig: Barth; 1910.

[9] Rabinovici G, Jagust W, Furst A, Ogar J, Racine C, Mormino E. Abeta amyloid and glucose metabolism in three variants of primary progressive aphasia. Annals of Neurology. 2008; 64: 388–401. DOI: 10.1002/ana.21451.

[10] Tang-Wai, D, Graff-Radford, N, Boeve, B, Dickson, D, Parisi, J, Crook, R. Clinical, genetic and neuropathologic characteristics of posterior cortical atrophy. Neurology. 2004; 63: 1168–1174. DOI: 10.1212/01.WNL.0000140289.18472.15.

[11] Clarfield A. The decreasing prevalence of reversible dementias: an updated meta-analysis. Archives of Internal Medicine. 2003; 163: 2219–2229. DOI: 10.1001/archinte.163.18.2219.

[12] Neary D. Non Alzheimer's disease forms of cerebral atrophy. Journal of Neurology and Neurosurgical Psychiatry. 1990; 53: 929–931. DOI: 10.1136/jnnp.53.11.929.

[13] Mesulam M. Slowly progressive aphasia without generalized dementia. Annals of Neurology, 1982; 11: 592–598. DOI: 10.1002/ana.410110607.

[14] Gorno-Tempini M, Hillis A, Weintraub S, Kertesz A, Mendez M, Cappa S, et al. Classification of primary progressive aphasia and its variants. Neurology. 2001; 76(11): 1006–1014. DOI: 10.1212/WNL.0b013e31821103e6.

[15] Alladi S, Xuereb J, Bak T, Nestor P, Knibb J, Patterson K, et al. Focal cortical presentations of Alzheimer's disease. Brain. 2006; 130: 2636–2645. DOI: 10.1093/brain/awm213.

[16] Knopman D, Parisi J, Salviati A, Floriach-Robert M, Boeve B, Ivnik R. Neuropathology of cognitively normal elderly. Journal of Neuropathology and Experimental Neuropsychology. 2003; 62: 1087–1089. DOI: 10.1093/jnen/62.11.1087.

[17] Prince J, Morris J. Tangles and plaques in nondemented aging and "preclinical" Alzheimer's disease. Annals of Neurology. 1999; 45: 358–368.

[18] Khachaturian Z. Diagnosis of Alzheimer's Disease. Archives of Neurology. 1985; 42; 1097–1105. DOI: 10.1001/archneur.1985.04060100083029.

[19] Mirra S, Heyman A, McKeel D, Sumi D, Crain B, Brownlee L. The Consortium to Establish a Registry for Alzheimer's Disease (CERAD). Part II. Standardization of the neuropathologic assessment of Alzheimer's disease. Neurology. 1991; 41: 479–486. DOI: 10.1212/WNL.41.4.479.

[20] Hayman B. The neuropathological diagnosis of Alzheimer's disease: clinical-pathological studies. Neurobiology of Aging. 1997; 18(4 Suppl.): S27–S32. DOI: 10.1016/S0197-4580(97)00066-3.

[21] Carrasco MM. Enfermedad de Alzheimer. In Agüera L, Cervilla J, Martín M, editors. Psiquiatría Geriátrica. Barcelona: Elsevier—Masson. 2006, pp. 184–208

[22] Clark C, Karlawish J. Alzheimer's disease: current concepts and emerging diagnostic and therapeutic strategies. Annals of Internal Medicine. 2001; 138: 400–410.

[23] Petersen R, Doody R, Kurz A, Mohs R, Morris J, Rabins P. et al. Current concepts in mild cognitive impairment. Archives of Neurology. 2001; 58: 1985–1992. DOI: 10.1001/archneur.58.12.1985

[24] Bruna O, Pelegrín C, Bartrés D, Gramunt N, Subirana J, Dergham A. Deterioro Cognitivo Leve [Mild Cognitive Impairment]. In: Bruna O, Roig T, Puyuelo M, Junqué C, Ruano A, editors. Rehabilitación neuropsicológica [Neuropsychological rehabilitation]. Barcelona: Elsevier—Masson; 2011. pp. 269–288.

[25] Petersen R, Smith G, Waring S, Ivnik R, Tangalos E, Kokmen E. Mild cognitive impairment: clinical characterization and outcome. Archives of Neurology. 1999; 56: 303–308. DOI: 10.1001/archneur.56.3.303.

[26] Flicker C, Ferris S, Reisberg B. Mild cognitive impairment in the elderly: predictors of dementia. Neurology. 1991; 41: 1006–1009. DOI: 10.1212/WNL.41.7.1006.

[27] Reisberg B, Ferris S, De Leon M, Crook, T. The Global Deterioration Scale for assessment of primary degenerative dementia. American Journal of Psychiatry. 1982; 139: 1136–1139.

[28] Sánchez-Rodríguez J, Torrellas-Morales C. Revisión del constructo de Deterioro Cognitivo Leve: aspectos generales [Review of the construct of Mild Cognitive Impairment: General Aspects]. Revista de Neurología. 2011; 52: 300–305.

[29] Albert M, DeKosky S, Dickson D, Dubois B, Feldman H, Fox, N, et al. (2011). The diagnosis of mild cognitive impairment due to Alzheimer's disease: recommendations from the National Institute on Aging and Alzheimer's Association workgroup. Alzheimer's & Dementia, 7(3): 270–279. DOI: 10.1016/j.jalz.2011.03.008.

[30] Busse A, Hensel A, Gühne U, Angermeyer M, Riedel-Heller S. Mild cognitive impairment: long-term course of four clinical subtypes. Neurology; 2006, 67(12): 2176–2185. DOI: 10.1212/01.wnl.0000249117.23318.e1.

[31] Nelson A, O'Connor M. Mild cognitive impairment: a neuropsychological perspective. CNS Spectrums. 2008; 13: 56–64.

[32] Sperling R, Aisen P, Beckett L, Bennet D, Craft S, Fagan A, et al. Toward defining the preclinical stages of Alzheimer's disease: recommendations from the National Institute

on Aging and the Alzheimer's Association workgroup. Alzheimer's & Dementia. 2011; 7(3): 280–292. DOI: 10.1016/j.jalz.2011.05.2351.

[33] Molinuevo J, Peña-Casanova J. Guía oficial para la práctica clínica en demencias: conceptos, criterios y recomendaciones [Official guide for clinical practice in dementias: concepts, criteria and recommendations]. Barcelona: Thomson Reuters; 2009.

[34] Levy R. Aging-associated cognitive decline. Working Party of the International Psychogeriatric Association in collaboration with the World Health Organization. International Psychogeriatrics. 1994; 6: 63–68. DOI: 10.1017/S1041610294001626.

[35] Winblad B, Palmer K, Kivipelto M, Jelic V, Fratiglioni L, Wahlund L, et al. Mild cognitive impairment beyond controversies, towards a consensus: report of the International Working Group on Mild Cognitive Impairment. Journal of Internal Medicine. 2004; 256(3): 240–246. DOI: 10.1111/j.1365-2796.2004.01380.x.

[36] Gauthier S, Touchon J. Subclasificación del deterioro cognitivo leve en las investigaciones y la práctica clínica [Sub-classification of mild cognitive impairment in research and clinical practice]. In Gauthier S, Sheltens P, Cummings J. Enfermedad de Alzheimer y trastornos relacionados. Barcelona: Ars Medica. 2006.

[37] Manly J, Tang M, Schupf N, Stern Y, Vonsattel J, Mayeux R. Frequency and course of mild cognitive impairment in a multiethnic community. Annals of Neurology. 2008; 63; 494–506. DOI: 10.1002/ana.21326.

[38] Ward A, Arright M, Michels S, Cedarbaum J. Mild cognitive impairment: disparity of incidence and prevalence estimates. Alzheimer's & Dementia. 2012; 8: 14–21. DOI: 10.1016/j.jalz.2011.01.002.

[39] Graham J, Rockwood D, Beattie L, Eastwood R, Gauthier S, Tuokko H, et al. Prevalence and severity of cognitive impairment with and without dementia in an elderly population. Lancet. 1997; 349: 1793–1796. DOI: 10.1016/S0140-6736(97)01007-6.

[40] Bennett D, Wilson R, Schneider J, Evans D, Beckett L, Aggarwal N. Natural history of mild cognitive impairment in older persons. Neurology. 2002; 59: 198–205. DOI: 10.1212/WNL.59.2.198.

[41] Jack C, Albert M, Knopman D, McKhann G, Sperling R, Carrillo M, et al. Introduction to the recommendations from the National Institute on Aging and the Alzheimer's Association workgroup on diagnostic guidelines for Alzheimer's disease. Alzheimer's & Dementia. 2011; 7(3): 257–262. DOI: 10.1016/j.jalz.2011.03.004.

[42] Setó-Salvia N, Clarimón J. Genética de la enfermedad de Alzheimer [Genetics of Alzheimer's disease]. Revista de Neurología. 2010; 50: 360–364.

[43] Guerreiro RJ, Gustafson DR, Hardy J. The genetic architecture of Alzheimer's disease: Beyond APP, PSENs and APOE, Neurobiology of Aging. 2012; 33(3): 437–456. DOI. 10.1016/j.neurobiolaging.2010.03.025.

[44] Van Duijn CM, Hofman A. Risk factors for Alzheimer's disease: the EURODEM collaborative re-analysis of case–control studies. Neuroepidemiology. 1992; 11 (Suppl 1): S106–S113. DOI: 10.1159/000111000.

[45] Bertam L, Lill C, Tanzi R. The genetics of Alzheimer disease: Back to the future. Neuron. 2010; 21: 270–281.

[46] Hardy J, Higgins G. Alzheimer's disease: the amyloid cascade hypothesis. Science. 1992; 256: 184–185. DOI: 10.1126/science.1566067.

[47] Selkoe D. Alzheimer's Disease. Cold Spring Harbor Perspectives in Biology. 2011; 3(7): 1–16. DOI:10.1101/cshperspect.a004457.

[48] Hardy J, Selkoe D. The amyloid hypothesis of Alzheimer's disease: progress and problems on the road to therapeutics. Science. 2002; 297: 353–356. DOI: 10.1126/science.1072994.

[49] Selkoe D. Defining molecular targets to prevent Alzheimer's disease. Archives of Neurology. 2005; 62: 192–195. DOI: 10.1001/archneur.62.2.192.

[50] Fagan A, Intun M, Mach R, Lee S, Dence C, Shah A. Inverse relation between in vivo amyloid imaging load and cerebrospinal fluid Abeta42 in humans. Annals of Neurology. 2006; 59: 512–519. DOI: 10.1002/ana.20730.

[51] Hampel H, Frank R, Broich K, Teipel S, Katz R, Herholtz K. Biomarkers for Alzheimer's disease: academic, industry and regulatory perspectives. Nature Reviews Drug Discovery. 2010; 9: 560–574. DOI: 10.1038/nrd3115.

[52] Kennard C. 2012. Biomarkers for Alzheimer's disease. Retrieved on 4 February 2012 from http://alzheimers.about.com/od/diagnosisissues/a/Biomarkers_Alz.htm.

[53] Bondi MW, Jak AJ, Delano-Wood L, Jacobson MW, Delis DC, Salmon DP. Neuropsychological contributions to the early identification of Alzheimer's disease. Neuropsychology Review. 2008; 18(1): 73–90. DOI: 10.1007/s11065-008-9054-1.

[54] Fratiglioni L, Wang HX. Brain reserve hypothesis in dementia. Journal of Alzheimer's Disease. 2009; 12: 11–22.

[55] Kawas CH, Katzman R. Epidemiology of dementia and Alzheimer's disease. In Terry RD, Bick KL, Sisodia SS, editors. Alzheimer's disease. 2nd ed. Lippincott Williams & Wilkins: Philadelphia. 1999, p. 95–116.

[56] Barnes DE, Yaffe K, Satariano WA, Tager IB. A longitudinal study of cardiorespiratory fitness and cognitive function in healthy older adults. Journal of the American Geriatrics Society. 2003; 15(10): 459–465. DOI: 10.1046/j.1532-5415.2003.51153.x.

[57] Kramer AF, Erickson KI. Capitalizing on cortical plasticity: influence of physical activity on cognition and brain function. Trends in Cognitive Sciences. 2007; 11(8): 342–348. DOI: 10.1016/j.tics.2007.06.009.

[58] Blessed G, Tomlinson BE, Roth, M. The association between quantitative measures of dementia and of senile change in the cerebral grey matter of elderly subjects. British Journal of Psychiatry. 1968; 114: 797–811. DOI: 10.1192/bjp.114.512.797.

[59] De la Torre JC. Alzheimer disease as vascular disorder: nosological evidence. Stroke. 2002; 33(4), 1152–1162. DOI: 10.1161/01.STR.0000014421.15948.67.

[60] Borenstein AR, Copenhaver CI, Mortimer JA. Early-life risk factors for Alzheimer disease. Alzheimer Disease and Associated Disorders. 2006; 20: 63–72. DOI: 10.1097/01.wad.0000201854.62116.d7.

[61] Carnero C, del Ser T. La educación proporciona reserva cognitiva en el deterioro cognitivo y la demencia [Education provides cognitive reserve in cognitive impairment and dementia].